Managing Herpes

D0731685

ISBN: 978-0-9814695-1-5
Copyright: © 2007 Standard Copyright License
Language: English
Country: United States

Table of Content

Introduction

There is no new cure. There is no permanent solution yet at hand. So why write yet another edition of this book? The chief objectives have not changed. There is a lot to know about having herpes, and the chapters to follow tell all. Since the last edition, there has been an explosion of discovery and new information around the subject. Much of the new information is reassuring and some a bit unsettling. A new technology called polymerase chain reaction (PCR) allows scientists to detect minute quantities of viral DNA from skin swabs. PCR studies of patients with recurrent genital herpes have shown that herpes probably reactivates far more frequently than anyone realized previously. On the other hand, the vast majority of these reactivations are promptly dealt with by the body's own immune system without ever allowing the viral shedding or clinical symptoms to take hold. Clinical studies have also now shown that safe, long-term recurrence reduction is possible. Proper use of medication can drastically reduce both symptomatic and asymptomatic viral shedding. Reducing asymptomatic shedding might also diminish the chances of asymptomatic transmission of herpes simplex virus, although this remains to be proven. Early results suggest that cesarean section might be avoidable in many cases by using acyclovir suppression during the last few weeks of pregnancy (see discussion chapter 6). Antiviral chemotherapy has reached its second generation and studies are under way to determine how much improvement we can identify. Dosing of treatments has become easier, and effectiveness has also improved. Vaccine trials for both prevention and treatment are ongoing although early results with one of the current vaccine candidates have been discouraging. The key issues for most people, though, remain the simple, personal ones. How do I tell my partner I have herpes? How do I avoid transmitting the infection? How do I break this burden of selfimposed secrecy and keep my self-esteem intact? How do I avoid feeling like a victim? How do I get on with my life?

Herpes has also changed over the past decade because of the AIDS epidemic. Research into HIV infection has brought with it new understanding of and new treatments for other viral diseases like herpes. The immune surveillance system that controls herpes in the normal host is diminished in AIDS, so herpes is one of the common problems affecting people with AIDS. But the AIDS epidemic has also meant that safer sex is becoming commonplace. If you are having sexual contact, you should be using safer sex practices. The sad truth, though, is that too many people are still not discussing safer sex or routinely practicing it. Safer sex practices should be considered the normal and usual thing to do until you and your partner have both determined your risks for all STDs including AIDS and until you have both decided to be completely monogamous. New data on genital herpes are also showing that safer sex in conjunction with avoiding intercourse altogether during active phases of infections is the best way to go for herpes prevention.

The past five years have provided lots of new information about the prevention of sexually transmitted herpes and also lots of new information about the prevention of herpes in newborn babies. Acyclovir has now been in general use for nearly fifteen years, and its safety has been remarkable, to date. Under certain circumstances, some physicians have even begun to prescribe acyclovir for chronic suppression in children and pregnant women (see discussion chapter 6). Two new drugs for herpes have been approved by the FDA. New drugs have a major role to play in the treatment of genital herpes. In some cases, though, drug treatment is not very helpful. The right drug used the wrong way can make coping with genital herpes more difficult. This book will help you and your physician through the maze of therapeutic decision-making.

The next generation of drugs for herpes may hold even more promise, and clinical trials are not far off. Scientists have identified some of the gene products of herpes that somehow allow the virus

to maintain its latent state. Certain genes allow herpes to become latent, stay latent and not reactivate at all. It is possible, therefore, that specific targets for new chemotherapy will be identified to attempt to prevent reactivation. Today, such products remain on the preclinical drawing boards. Ten years ago, however, there were no such discussions. Ten years from now, new treatments and vaccines willlikely be preventing new infection in partners and reducing the problem of herpes recurrences even further. Reversing genetic characteristics of latent herpes to prevent further disease could well be the next step.

Hopes for cures remain alive. In the meantime, new discoveries and old discoveries make treatments much more safe and effective. Use them wisely. You don't need to become celibate or promiscuous in an effort to cope with herpes. Instead, you can stress honesty and be selective in choosing partners on the basis of mutual respect. You can use safer sex practices to avoid the transmission of AIDS, Chlamydia, papillomavirus, gonorrhea, and herpes. You can talk about your herpes assertively and apologize to no one for being clear about what is going on in your own body and for knowing what to do about it. Especially, you don't need to apologize to yourself. You can find out what you need to find out, discuss what you need to discuss, and treat what you need to treat. This book should help you to do all three.

The Most Important Questions First

Am I contagious between recurrences? Do I have to give up sex?

Medical explanations of herpes are given in the forthcoming chapters. For now, it is most important to know that the virus called *herpes simplex* can exist in two very different states: active, in which the virus is growing on the skin, often forming lesions, and latent, in which the virus is dormant within the nervous system, causing no harm. The latent period is a quiet period that persists for life. From the latent state, the herpes virus may seed a recurrence of an active skin infection.

When your herpes is in the latent state, there is no virus on your skin and you cannot infect your sexual partner. Herpes is only transmitted when active virus on the skin comes into direct contact with the skin of another person who is susceptible. But it is not always possible to know when the virus has reactivated-some infections can go entirely unnoticed. Therefore people with herpes should avoid sore-to-skin contact when obvious skin lesions are present and safer sex should be practiced between episodes-just in case the virus has reactivated without being recognized.

People with herpes must get to know their own recurrence pattern and learn the skills necessary to identify the active periods when the virus is on the skin (see chapter 3). They can then adjust their sexual activity around these times, avoiding sore-to-skin contact during the active phases. Active phases are not made safe by covering a sore with a latex condom.

Often, active herpes infections are mild and not especially bothersome. Every so often, most people with herpes have outbreaks so mild that nothing at all is detected. This no symptoms/no signs recurrence on the skin is called *asymptomatic shedding-a* period of virus reactivation so mild that sores are not detected. A swab taken from the affected area at that time and sent to the laboratory, though, would show that herpes is actively growing on the skin. Thus, it is possible to transmit herpes even though you cannot see a lesion. New data show that suppressive use of antiviral medication-taken continuously twice a day-may reduce the risk of asymptomatic shedding by about 80 percent. Even though asymptomatic shedding occurs less than 5 percent of the time, a person with herpes who is partnered with someone who does not have herpes can take one additional and very effective step toward reducing the risk of transmission: safer sexual practices. The consistent use of latex condoms to prevent direct skin contact during the latent state markedly reduces the chance that an unrecognized recurrence might lead to transmission. In addition, people with herpes should get to know the facts about herpes, so that they can inform their partners assertively and comfortably and be able to explain the risks. Limiting contact to others who have the same infection would accomplish nothing. Furthermore, celibacy would do the world no favor. Indeed, in the long run these extreme measures would do a great deal of harm, both to individuals with herpes and to society at large.

My spouse is my only sexual partner. We've been together for months and I just got herpes. Is my spouse to blame? Has my spouse been unfaithful?

Genital herpes is a sexually transmitted disease. In theory, there is a small possibility of obtaining the infection from another sourcefor instance, from a warm, moist towel that someone else has just used. In practice, however, for the virus to affect the genitals it must be put *onto* the genitals, and the best way of doing that is via sex. Herpes infections flare up and then heal in a very short cycle, so the virus becomes active, then latent, and then active again. Also, *most* people with genital herpes do not know they have it and never have any symptoms that they identify. Your partner could have been infected in the past and may have had sex with you at the exact moment that he or she had an active infection. There is also the possibility that you have had genital herpes for several years and only just now noticed symptoms. Only very sophisticated laboratory tests can tell the difference between primary and recurrent herpes.

If you have oral sex while either you or your partner are actively shedding virus from the lips or mouth, genital herpes may result. For example, if your partner's mouth came into contact with your genitals, you may have been infected with genital herpes. This can happen if your partner had an active cold sore, a fever blister, or a mouth sore caused by the herpes virus-or even if he or she had no recognized symptoms at all. In fact, 50 to 80 percent of people harbor the virus in a latent state and shed the virus in the mouth during recurrences of active infection.

Herpes simplex causes both mouth and genital herpes. The mouth type of herpes infection is usually caused by *herpes simplex virus type J,* and is most often spread from mouth to mouth (and often from parent to child). Genital herpes is usually caused by *herpes simplex virus type* 2. However, there is no hard and fast rule about this. While type 1 likes the mouth best and type 2   likes the genitals best, the virus can be transmitted from a site on one person's body to another site on the partner's body, depending on what body part contacts what. (If the virus is on the toe and if the toe spends a lot of time in someone else's ear, an infection in his or her ear can result.) The viral type does not change when the site of infection changes. If you received genital herpes from a type 1 herpes simplex cold sore on your partner, your genital herpes sores will still be type 1. There is no change of the virus type when it now appears on the genital skin. So your partner could have received herpes of the mouth from a parent at age three, have had no symptoms, and still have transmitted the virus to your genitals thirty years later!

So be careful before calling the divorce lawyer. Talk the problem out with your partner. Don't let herpes alone come between you. Be honest and demand honesty. Possibly your partner was with another partner and your genital herpes was the first sign-but possibly not. An honest discussion about herpes may even bring you closer together.

Herpes of the newborn is a deforming, blinding, often fatal disease. Should I give up my plans to have children?

No. Since herpes is spread from active skin infection and not from latent infection, a newborn baby can be infected with herpes only if he or she is born while the virus is active. *Neonatal herpes* generally occurs if the baby's skin becomes infected during the birth process. If herpes is latent in the mother, there is no virus along the birth canal to infect the baby. If herpes sores are present at the time of labor, then (and only then) a cesarean section may be required to reduce the possibility of direct contact between the infection and the baby. Before birth, the membranes surrounding the baby are a natural barrier that helps to prevent the virus from travelling from the mother's skin to the baby's skin. If the membranes rupture (the bag of water breaks) and a herpes sore on or near the vagina is active, a cesarean section is often performed as an emergency operation. If no sores are present, however, normal labor may safely proceed. Many centers are now studying the use of regular oral acyclovir during the last two to four weeks of pregnancy to prevent reactivations and allow for a normal vaginal delivery. You may wish to discuss this with your doctor.

In order to avoid giving herpes to your baby, you must also tell your doctor that you have herpes (or that a previous partner had or your present partner has herpes). During labor, the doctor will carefully inspect your genitals, especially the external genital area, for herpes sores. You must take an active role and discuss the problem well in advance with your doctor. Regular, careful examinations of the external genitals by your physician during the last two or three weeks of pregnancy may be useful, depending upon how frequently you get recurrences. You and the doctor should increase your awareness of your herpes outbreaks-what they feel like, what they look like, and so on. If possible, your doctor will take a herpes culture from the skin around the vagina during labor; in the unlikely event that a sore has been missed, there will be time to watch and treat the baby, if necessary. The chances that a mother with recurrent genital herpes will give birth to a baby who becomes ill with neonatal herpes are only about one in several thousands, as long as you and your doctor are aware of the status of your infection and are attuned to prevention.

A fetus can also get a herpes infection *inside* the womb. In this situation, herpes could have a harmful effect on the fetus before birth. This syndrome of *congenital herpes* is very rare. Some physicians believe that *primary herpes* (the first episode of herpes) in the mother may lead to infection in the womb, especially if primary herpes occurs in early pregnancy. However, the overwhelming majority of women who have primary herpes during the first two trimesters of pregnancy give birth to perfectly normal babies. Primary herpes in early pregnancy is not considered an absolute indication for abortion, although some women in this situation may choose to have abortions. One study from Seattle showed that one in five such situations (true primary herpes in the first trimester of pregnancy) led to a miscarriage where the fetus was shown to have been affected by herpes in the uterus. Because this situation is so uncommon, the study may have underestimated or overestimated the true incidence. Follow-up unpublished studies from the same medical center suggest that one in five may be an overestimate. Nothing specific can be done to prevent congenital herpes, but the risk is very low. In fact, even women with a proven herpes infection inside the womb often have completely normal and unaffected babies. Most healthy and well-nourished babies who are born to women with herpes are very unlikely to develop problems.

When you consider how many new mothers have had a genital herpes infection, it may seem surprising that herpes of the newborn remains an uncommon disease. Some physicians believe that antibodies account for this low incidence. Most people with herpes make plenty of herpes antibodies-proteins that neutralize the virus on contact (see chapter 2). The antibodies probably get into the amniotic fluid in which the baby floats, coating the baby in a layer of protection. Antibodies may knock out the virus before (or after) it gets onto the baby's skin. The exact role of protective antibodies is not fully known. However, we do know that compared with recurrent genital herpes in the mother, primary genital herpes during late pregnancy (where antibodies are not yet available) results in a much greater risk to the newborn baby. Neonatal herpes is very uncommon, while recurrent genital herpes in pregnancy is extremely common.

Recent studies by Charles Prober and Ann Arvin at Stanford University have focused on primary infection as a risk for neonatal herpes. They have looked specifically at women in the third trimester of their pregnancy who do not have any antibodies to herpes and who are susceptible to primary type 2 genital herpes because their partners have type 2 genital herpes. This "discordance of pairs" is a specific situation in which a pregnant woman could be expected to develop a primary infection. The data show that women with true primary infections are at much greater risk of transmitting their infection to their babies than are women with recurrent infections.

Another way to look at this is that if a pregnant woman knows she has herpes and has had it for awhile, she is protected by nature from transmitting herpes to the newborn in most cases. Her baby acquires immunity to herpes from her. If she sheds virus asymptomati cally, her baby will probably be exposed, if at all, to only a small amount of virus, which will probably be readily neutralized by her immunity. If, on the other hand, the baby is exposed to a primary infection, a large amount of virus is present, often on the cervix, and the pregnant woman has not yet developed protective antibodies. That is the really dangerous situation. Recurrent herpes in the pregnant woman, which is more common, is usually less problematic. In fact, some epidemiologists feel that there is a significantly greater threat to the mother from having a cesarean than there is to the infant who might be exposed to a recurrent lesion. This is still controversial, but it does point to the fact that part of the problem with herpes in pregnancy is the number of unnecessary cesareans performed. There are exceptions to everything, of course, but it is OK to get pregnant and have a baby even though you or your partner have herpes. If you are pregnant and your sexual partner has herpes and you don't, then you should be very careful. Follow all safe sexual practices during the first two trimesters and especially during the third trimester. In fact, it is safest in this situation to avoid sexual contact during the third trimester. Do not avoid getting pregnant because of herpes, but do take time to understand the issues.

Can herpes cause cancer?

Does herpes infection lead to cancer? Several years ago, investigators noticed that people with more active sex lives had a statistically higher chance of getting cancer of the cervix. Celibacy, then, is one way to avoid cervical cancer. In fact, this cancer almost never occurs in Catholic nuns. There is no question that sex causes cervical cancer. Herpes antibodies are much more likely to be present in blood samples from women with cervical cancer than in blood samples from women without this cancer. Does this prove that herpes caused the cancer-or does it only show that herpes relates to sexual activity and that something else about sexual activity relates to cervical cancer? Herpes does not seem to cause cervical cancer. Human papillomavirus, which causes genital warts, is now receiving the most attention in research into cervical cancer. Certain subtypes of this virus appear to be the main causes of cervical cancer. As the evidence mounts for papillomavirus as a cause, the association between herpes and cervical cancer is rapidly diminishing.

Regardless of the possible causes of cervical cancer, every woman can take steps to prevent complications of this easily detected cancer. Happily, cervical cancer grows very slowly at first and is easy to detect in its early stages. Cure is virtually guaranteed if cervical cancer is detected early. Major surgery is generally not required to halt the disease in the early stages. Easy detection is accomplished by the *Papanicolaou (Pap) smear*. I recommend that women with herpes have annual Pap smears-not only as a precaution but also for peace of mind. The Pap test is a quick, simple, and painless test that samples the coating on the cervix (the mouth of the womb). Under the microscope, cancer cells in the specimen can be detected in their earliest stage.

All women should have this test done regularly, and women who have had herpes or any sexually transmitted disease should have it done at least once a year. Beyond a regular Pap test, no other precautions against cervical cancer are necessary.

Conclusion

Herpes is able to cause a recurrent skin infection. People most often remain totally unaware that they have this infection. However, once herpes has been diagnosed, its recurrence can usually be clearly recognized. Avoiding transmission comes

13

naturally once you understand the active phases of infection and begin to use safer sex practices. Control of your infection comes gradually as your own army of immunity takes over and fights off each recurrence with efficient killing power. With time, the frequency of recurrences may diminish. The virus may cause a terrible infection in some newborn babies, but this syndrome tends to occur most commonly where the mother is experiencing her first-ever (primary) genital infection. Mothers with recurrent genital herpes are largely protected from this complication by their own immunity, which is passed on to the child more efficiently than the virus itself. Neonatal herpes is a highly preventable and uncommon disease, and it is almost always under the control of the mother and her physician if she knows she has herpes and discusses the problem.

Cervical cancer, which is probably caused by human papillomavirus, is statistically associated with herpes as well. It is highly doubtful that herpes actually causes this cancer. Through the yearly Pap smear, this cancer can be easily detected and effectively dealt with. It is unlikely to occur, herpes or no herpes.

Is herpes an incurable disease that kills babies and causes cervical cancer? No. On the contrary, herpes is an extremely common virus infection, poorly understood by many people and further sensationalized by the media. It is a nuisance, without doubt. It can be a problem when it recurs very frequently. Safe and effective drug therapy that reduces the frequency of both symptomatic and asymptomatic recurrences is now available. Herpes can sometimes result in serious complications, but people who have herpes can easily prevent these complications. If you have the right information, herpes is a syndrome that can be under your control.

Herpes Simplex: The Virus

A short history of herpes

Herpes infections are not new. Over twenty-five centuries ago Hippocrates, the father of medicine, coined the word "herpes" from the Greek "to creep." Medicine in his time was descriptive; diseases were classified according to their appearance. The diseases that Hippocrates called herpes are now known to be several different skin maladies with several different names and causes.

In the first part of this century, scientists discovered the "filterable virus," a particle so small that it could pass through a paper filter and could not be seen with the microscope and yet was fully capable of causing infection. It was not long before microbiologists had identified many different viruses capable of causing different diseases. Some examples are polio, hepatitis, influenza, and rhinovirus (the common cold). The virus that causes herpes was identified as herpes simplex. The cause of herpes infections became further understood and the different kinds of herpes viruses further classified.

A great step forward in understanding viruses was the development of the technology for growing viruses outside the body-Le., in vitro (in the test tube). Since viruses are parasites of cells, they need cells in which to grow. The first advance in the field was the discovery that human cells could be stimulated to grow artificially by giving them the right nutrients and keeping them at the right temperature. Cells are the "unit system" of the body. They contain all the parts necessary for reproduction and metabolism; that is, they can make new copies of themselves and carry out the chemical processes needed for life. Furthermore, each type of cell in the body has a special function. **It** might specialize in moving body parts (muscle cells), building structures (bone cells), filtering out poison (kidney cells), detoxifying poison (liver cells), guarding the body surface (epithelial cells), killing foreign invaders (lymphocytes and leukocytes), or carrying oxygen to other cells (erythrocytes).

Pick any organ or system of the body-whether it be for pumping blood or for thinking. If you look at a slice of this tissue under the microscope, you will see different cells, each doing its thing. Figure 1 is from such a slice of normal skin. The cells can be seen lined up according to function. The epithelial cells are the special targets of the herpes simplex virus. Note the thick layer of keratin, a waxy outer coating of skin that forms a natural physical barrier to ward off invasion by infection.

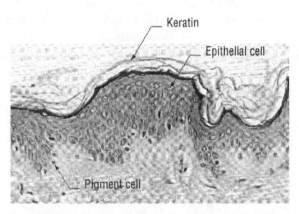

Figure I: A microscope view of a slice of skin. As long as the waxy outer coating of keratin stays unbroken, it helps to prevent herpes simplex virus from finding its target-
the epithelial (skin) cells. The cells with the dark pigment (called melanin) give the skin its color.

16

Viruses are grown in the laboratory by allowing them to infect normal body cells growing in the test tube. First the body cells must be grown in culture. To do this, a piece of tissue is placed in a test tube with chemicals and enzymes and carefully chopped up. The separated cells are then given nutrients like sugar, amino acids, and vitamins. If everything goes well, the cells will soon grow and multiply. Figure 2 shows skin cells grown in culture. No longer specialized for skin, these cells are all of the same type, called fibroblasts.

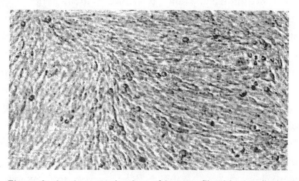

Figure 2: A microscopic view of human fibroblast cells grown in tissue culture. Cells in the laboratory look like this if they are healthy-not affected by a virus or anything else. Different viruses can be detected by the changes they induce in these cells.

Once scientists were able to grow cells in vitro (outside the body), getting viruses to grow inside those cells became easier. Viruses were soon purified, analyzed, and classified. Herpes simplex virus could be detected from sores, on the genitals and elsewhere. At first, herpes was not considered to be a sexually transmitted disease. It was later shown, however, that the greater the number of sexual partners an individual had, the greater the risk of contracting herpes.

By the late 1960s, herpes of the newborn had been linked to an active herpes infection in the mother at the time of birth. This marked the beginning of an explosive period of herpes research.

Cervical cancer was (erroneously) connected with herpes. As more became known about herpes, it became more widely publicized, and the public alarm made good press. More people with bothersome sores sought medical help. At the same time, the population became more sexually active. Society loosened many sexual taboos. Casual sexual contact and oral sex became more frequent. Possibly the most important factor in increasing herpes, however, was the change of birth control methods. As people left behind condoms and foam for the convenience of the IUD and the pill, they left behind effective barriers to infection.

Today, we have a reservoir of virus in the community that is so large that herpes has become almost unavoidable. Today, ten times as many people seek help from a physician for genital herpes as they did twenty years ago. Studies in Vancouver, British Columbia, show that 20 percent of women who have ever had sex have genital herpes type 2. Once they have had six or more sexual partners, about 40 percent of women have genital herpes. Having had more than ten sexual partners gives women a risk of almost 60 percent for genital herpes. Studies in African-American populations show that men have an incidence of about 40 percent and women an incidence of about 60 percent. In all studies and all populations, men have a slightly lower risk of acquiring genital herpes. Their different anatomy seems to make them slightly less likely to get herpes from a partner. Yet both sexes are at significantly high risk-a risk that is not related to their exposure to partners who are known to have herpes. Consistent use of safer sex practice will lower the risks, but unfortunately, most couples do not use them. You don't have to be a statistician to see the problem we face now and in the future.

What is a virus, anyway?

A virus is a very small living thing. It is so small that it can pass through something as fine as a coffee filter. It cannot live on its own. A virus contains either DNA or RNA (hereditary material that passes on characteristics to the next generation of viruses). As depicted in the graphic illustration (see plate 1, page 95), this hereditary material is surrounded by a protective coat made of protein and sometimes by another protective outer coat called an *envelope,* which is made of fatty and protein-like material. An electron micrograph of herpes is shown in figure 3.

A virus lives according to all known laws of heredity and natural selection. Its biological job is to make copies of itself, called *daughter particles.* A virus reproduces in a straightforward fashion. First, since it is a parasite, it seeks a host cell that provides a suitable environment. Each virus has its own favorite type of host cell. Which cell the virus likes best partly determines which disease it causes. For example, hepatitis viruses like liver cells, while herpes simplex viruses like skin and nerve cells.

Plate 2 shows how herpes infects an epithelial (skin) cell (see plate 2, page 96, simplified for clarity). After finding the cell, the virus attaches itself (probably to special receptors or receiving sites) to the outer layer of the cell, called the *membrane.* It then "undresses" itself and injects its hereditary material (DNA) into the cell. The DNA finds its way to the cell nucleus, where it uses the cell's own machinery to make virus daughter particles. Usually this reproduction of new viruses stops the host cell from living for itself. After new virus particles are made, the human cell bursts and dies, scattering daughter particles around to neighboring cells, where the cycle is repeated.

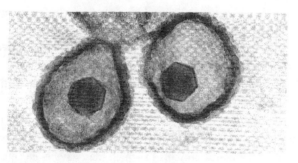

Figure 3: *An electron micrograph of two herpes simplex viruses. Note the highly organized geometric shape of the nucleocapsid surrounded by a large, shapeless envelope.*

Viruses have a different relationship with human cells than bacteria do. Bacteria are self-sufficient-living all on their own. A virus is a parasite; it survives by taking over the host cell machinery. That is why a virus is so hard to kill. Bacteria (gonorrhea, for example) don't need a host cell in which to live and grow. They are a part of the plant kingdom in nature and need only basic nutrients (carbohydrates, proteins, and so forth). Because bacteria can make so many of their own products, they are easy to kill with antibiotics (such as penicillin), which interrupt some manufacturing process that is vital to the bacteria but is of no concern to the human body. (penicillin, for example, interrupts the manufacture of the bacterial cell wall. It has no effect on human cells, because animal cells do not have a cell wall.) The virus needs its host cell, however, and since the virus uses the host cell's manufacturing system for its own life cycle, many chemicals that kill the virus also interrupt the normal host metabolism. That is why, to date, there is no cure for the common cold and no cure for herpes.

We are learning more and more about viruses, however. As researchers find things that viruses do that are unique to the virus, so are they able to find ways of killing the virus without harming the host. In fact, researchers can now use the special chemistry of herpes viruses to select and kill cancer cells. This is done by transferring parts of viral DNA to a cancerous tumor, using another virus as a vector, or carrier.

What stops a viral infection?

The growth cycle of a virus is eventually halted by the coordinated strategy of the body's immune system, which has two major components: the *humoral* system and *cell-mediated* system (see plate 15, page 102). The humoral system uses cells called lymphocytes to recognize viral glycoproteins. When triggered by these glycoproteins, the B lymphocytes produce proteins called antibodies. The antibodies cling to the virus particles and inactivate them. The cell-mediated component of the immune system uses fighter cells called T lymphocytes. T lymphocytes called CD8 cells (also called "cytotoxic" T cells) look around for infected cells that contain viral proteins to which they have been sensitized. When they find such a cell, they attack and kill it. CD4 cells (also called "helper" T cells) help by stimulating T cells and B cells to grow and do their jobs. CD4 cells are the main target of HIV, and their depletion causes many of the problems in AIDS patients whose cellmediated immunity is depleted.

Macrophages (see plate 5, page 97) then come along as janitors and clean up the mess, leaving room for healthy, unaffected cells to grow and replace the old.

Why don't we develop immunity to herpes? (The story of latent infection)

We really do develop immunity to herpes. The body's immune system is very effective at stopping a recurrence once it starts. But how, then, is it able to start at all? Herpes simplex has two tricks up its sleeve to beat the system. Although most of the virus is wiped out by the body's defenses, some virus finds its way up the nerve endings that give feeling to the affected areas of skin.

The body's sensory nervous network gives physical sensations such as pain, temperature sensation, and touch sensation. To accomplish this, nerve fibers extend to all areas of skin like a branching network of phone cables supplying many houses with phone service. Groups of nerve fibers gather up the electrical input from several areas into one cable for transmission to the brain and feed into their local switching station, called a *ganglion*. The ganglia lie next to the spinal cord-the main cable-and house the cell machinery for all the nerve fibers. There are several ganglia running along the spinal cord from top to bottom.

The herpes virus wastes no time in establishing its latent state, penetrating the nerve fiber (axon) very quickly after infecting the skin cell. The nucleocapsid (containing the DNA) travels up the nerve fiber and stops when it gets to the ganglion, shown in figure 4. In some of the nerve cells, the virus comes to rest; in others it proceeds with its active growth cycle. Herpes decides very quickly whether it will cause a latent or an active infection in each cell it infects. Why does it go to rest in some cells *(latent infection)* while growing actively *(productive infection)* in others? A dual infection system (latent and productive) gives the virus a strong persistence mechanism. Within the nerve cells identified for latent (dormant) infection, there appears to be no significant damage to

2.

the nerve. In fact, this infection state is so quiet that the body's defenses do not even sense a problem. While the body's immune system effectively eradicates active viral infection in the skin, it does not even try to put up a fight against latent infection in the nerve. Herpes is so effective at establishing itself in the latent state that, in laboratory tests, it seems to be able to become latent even if a genetic mutation prevents the virus from normal reproduction.

Figure 4: During active skin infection, while the infected epithelial cells are going through their battle with the immune system, it is thought that the nerve fibers that supply sensation to the affected areas of skin also become infected (lower box). The virus travels up the nerve fiber until it gets to the core of the cell inside the ganglion. There it stops. Unlike the productive and explosive infection occuring on the skin, infection of the nerve cell results in quiet, or latent, infection that persists (upper box).

Sacral Ganglion Herpes

Simplex Virus

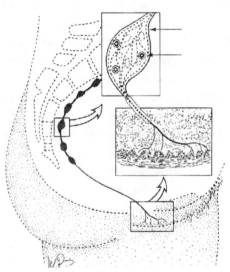

Several copies of the viral DNA are present inside each latently infected human nerve cell. It is not known whether this occurs because several virus particles attack a single cell or because one virus particle produces several latent copies of itself. Many nerve cells in an affected ganglion may be infected. The viral DNA exists inside the neuron in the form of circles that are extrachromosomal (not incorporated into the human host cell's DNA). This viral DNA is associated with cellular proteins called histones. From its latent state, virus can be cultivated from ganglion cells removed in autopsies, under very special conditions of care, called co *cultivation.* In the body, reactivation from latent to productive infection occurs from time to time. Reactivation can be induced by a neurosurgeon operating near a latently infected ganglion. In such a case, herpes recurs at the original skin site as a postoperative complication.

Inside the neuronal nucleus, herpes simplex virus makes a type of RNA known as a *latency-associated transcript,* or LAT. LATs are not actually required to ensure that latency occurs, although they do seem to make it easier for herpes to reactivate. Only some of the factors that determine latency of herpes simplex virus come from the virus, however. Many other factors that govern herpes simplex viral latency in neurons are controlled strictly by certain characteristics of the host nerve cell.

Every ganglion is different, and every person is different. On the face, type 1 herpes simplex virus tends to recur more than type 2 herpes simplex virus, because type 1 reactivates more efficiently from the trigeminal ganglia located near the brain stem. On the genitals and buttocks, type 2 tends to recur more than type 1, because type 2 reactivates more efficiently from the sacral ganglia, located near the base of the spine (figure 4). A strain of virus that reactivates infrequently in one person may reactivate frequently in another. Viral factors are important, such as the virulence of the specific viral strain, the quantity of virus infecting the person, the viral type (type 1 versus type 2) and other genetic factors of the virus and its heritage. Human host factors include the susceptibility of the infected person as determined by heredity and immunity, whether or not there has been previous exposure to another strain of herpes simplex virus, and the length of exposure to the virus. Latent virus remains dormant holding the potential to reactivate when triggered to do so.

Latency: the reactivation process from sacral ganglia to genital skin
Herpes simplex virus follows a defined route upon reactivation. It travels down the nerve fibers that emanate from the speclflc nerve

cell that is reactivating. The cells harboring latent virus are logically in the ganglia where nerve fibers lead from the genital skin. In general, then, herpes travels back down nerve fibers in the same general vicinity as those first affected. After travelling back down to the end of the nerve fiber, the virus reaches the surface of a new, uninfected skin cell, attaches itself to receptors at the cell surface, and penetrates the healthy skin cell. Since nerve fibers tend to branch into related groups of smaller fibers, herpes often appears on the skin as a cluster of tiny sores, each representing the result of one virus particle recurring at one cell at the end of one tiny nerve fiber. Then, the active state begins again and a new recurrent infection takes place. The recurrent infection once again signals danger to the body's immune system, and the antibodies and cells go to work halting the active infection. Recurrences are often less severe than first-time skin infection, because neutralizing antibodies were made the first time. T lymphocytes were targeted and are already there, waiting to attack emerging *virions* (daughter virus particles). At the time of the first infection, if the first infection was truly primary, antibodies had not yet formed, and so lesions took longer to heal, affected more skin, and caused more blisters and symptoms. Now the immune system is able to halt the recurrence in short order. However, preventing the reactivation from beginning is not so easy, because the virus hibernates in a quiet or latent state in a nerve cell and then travels back to the skin via the inside of the nerve's fiber until the reactivation process has begun, thus sneaking by the body's immune system until the reactivation process has already been set in motion.

Remember, herpes has *two* tricks. The first is its ability to remain latent in the nerve cells. The second is its ability to go from one cell to another without ever leaving the cell environment. Suppose you decided to rob houses in your neighborhood by going from your house to your neighbor's house without ever going outdoors. In that way you could avoid the police. To go a step further, you could send a signal to a carpenter in your neighbor's house telling him or her to build a self-enclosed bridge to your house. This is exactly what herpes simplex virus does. The cell with virus fuses with its neighbor cell by inducing bridges. So many cells may fuse that a *multinucleated giant cell* is formed. (These giant cells are so specific for herpes that they are one way the virologist can tell if a virus culture is growing herpes.)

Why is this bridging important? With most viruses, immunity is a sufficient defense to prevent a recurrence. The basis for preventive vaccines like polio and measles is that the vaccine stimulates antibody production: when the virus comes along, it is neutralized by the antibodies before it spawns a disease. Since antibody is a very good virus poison, and since most viruses grow inside cells and then release themselves into the interstitial (extracellular) environment when the cell bursts, disease cannot recur. Antibodies are waiting, and the infection is nipped in the bud. Herpes is different. Most herpes-infected cells do burst, and most of the herpes virus is neutralized, but antibodies cannot easily travel to the inside of a cell to attack a virus-and herpes is busy building bridges *before* its growth has progressed to the cell-bursting stage. A few virions saunter happily to a neighboring cell, safely protected inside the cell. Other emerging young virions that break outside to the interstitial spaces will be killed effectively and quickly by neutralizing antibodies, but a select few stay inside cells and live on for a short time to infect healthy neighboring cells. Quite a trick! Of course, the immune system cuts this process off by using its lymphocytes and macrophages to identify infected cells and clear up the mess-just as our imaginary scheme for robbing houses would not get very far before the police put a stop to it.

Antibodies are very helpful in limiting the severity of herpes recurrences, but the immune system cannot prevent recurrences from reactivating entirely. Recent clinical studies with one of the new vaccine candidates (Chiron-Biocine) have, in fact, shown that boosting the immune system with that herpes vaccine does not reduce recurrence rates or prevent infections in partners. Vaccines may very well induce many kinds of immunity, including neutralizing antibodies and viral-specific immune cells. We know that the immune system naturally and effectively controls the severity of herpes infections. However, despite the best fight the immune system can muster, recurrences of herpes may reactivate as small sores before the body reacts to shut down the process.

Herpes is very effective at hiding from its enemies. Hippocrates chose a remarkably apt name for herpes-to creep.

What is a herpes virus?

The herpes family of viruses includes eight different viruses that affect human beings. The official names are known by numerical designation as *human herpes virus* 1 through 8 (HHVI-HHV8):

1. **Human herpes virus 1 (HHVI)** is the official name for *herpes simplex virus type* 1, discussed at length in this book. It can cause cold sores or herpes of the eye, and it commonly causes first episodes of genital herpes.

3. **Human herpes virus 2 (HHV2)** is the official name for *herpes simplex virus type* 2, the most common cause of genital herpes and, less frequently, herpes of the newborn. It is much less commonly associated with facial and eye infections.

4. **Human herpes virus 3 (HHV3)** is the official name for *herpes zoster virus* (also called *varicella zoster virus),* the cause of chickenpox. Like its close relative, herpes simplex virus, herpes zoster likes to infect skin cells and nerve cells. The first three human herpes viruses are called *neurotropic* (also called *"alpha")* because of their characteristic love for nerve cells. Chickenpox is the primary (first-time) infection with herpes zoster. This virus may also recur along nerve fiber pathways, causing multiple sores where nerve fibers end on skin cells. Because the entire ganglion tends to reactivate with this virus, the physical severity of a recurrence is generally much worse than a recurrence of herpes simplex virus. Recurrent varicella virus infection of the skin is commonly known as either *zoster* or *shingles.* Both words translate from different languages into "belt" which describes the pattern in which the lesions appear on the body. Shingles only occurs once (or, rarely, twice). If you are told that your frequently recurrent herpes infection is frequent herpes zoster or shingles infection, a misdiagnosis has probably been made; have this checked out carefully with a reliable virus test.

4. Human herpes virus 4 (HHV4) is the official name of *EpsteinBarr virus,* the major cause of infectious mononucleosis, or mono ("kissing disease").

5. Human herpes virus 5 (HHV5) is the official name of *cytomegalovirus* (CMV). CMY is also a cause of mono. It can be sexually transmitted, can cause problems to newborns, and can cause hepatitis. Occasionally it is transmitted by blood transfusion. It is very common among homosexual men and is often associated with (but is not the cause 00 AIDS. CMY infection is one of the most difficult complications of AIDS, often leading to severe visual problems or even blindness, infection of the gastrointestinal tract, diarrhea, and a variety of other difficult problems-even death. For a virus that barely causes a problem in most people with normal immunity, it can be amazingly nasty in people with severely compromised immunity.

6. Human herpes virus 6 (HHV6) is a recently observed agent found in the blood cells of a few patients with a variety of diseases. It is known to be the cause of roseola in small children and can also cause a variety of other illnesses associated with fever in that age group, even where the typical roseola rash is missing. This infection apparently accounts for many of the cases of convulsions associated with fever in infancy *(febrile seizures).*

7. Human herpes virus 7 (HHV7) is even more recently observed. Like all human herpes viruses, HHY6 and 7 are ubiquitous. In other words, they are so common that most of humankind has been infected at some point-usually early in life. It is not at all clear what clinical effects this virus causes.

8. Human herpes virus 8 (HHV8) was recently discovered in the tumors called *Kaposi's Sarcoma* (KS) that are found in people with AIDS (and are otherwise very rare). KS forms purplish tumors in the skin and other tissues of some people with AIDS and has been very difficult to treat with medication. HHY8 may also cause other cancers, including certain lymphomas associated with AIDS. The fact that these cancers are caused by a

virus may explain why such complications tend to occur in people with AIDS when their immune systems begin to fail. The discovery also provides new hope that specific treatments for these tumors will be developed that target the virus.

Genital Herpes: The Symptoms

What are the symptoms of genital herpes?

Herpes, like any other infection, causes a spectrum of symptoms from very mild to very severe. There are people whose lab tests prove they have had infection but who show no symptoms whatsoever, while, on the other hand, there are people whose symptoms are so severe that they result in extreme disability or even death. An example of the latter would be a newborn baby who became infected with herpes that disseminated throughout the body.

When it causes infection in a normal person, however, genital herpes almost never results in severe disability or death. Most people with genital herpes are at the opposite end of the spectrum. They have been exposed to genital herpes and have developed latent infection and antibodies but have never had any symptoms of active infection. It is difficult, then, to paint a single picture of what herpes infection is like. The symptoms depend not only on the severity of infection but also on its site, which in turn is largely determined by the site of inoculation. In other words, where did the herpes virus find its easiest access to epithelial cells of the skin? For the most part, herpes simplex prefers mucous membranes, where the skin is thin. These include areas like the labia (lips) of the vagina and the lips of the mouth. However, any area of the body may be fair territory for herpes. If a finger has a tiny crack on it (which it commonly does), any herpes simplex virus sitting on the finger can easily find its way to an epithelial cell. In general, though, it is difficult for the virus to enter the skin on the hand and other thick-skinned areas. However, any time there is excessive moisture, and especially if there is trauma or injury that compromises the normal protection of the area, the setting is ideal for herpes to be transmitted. (For further information on autoinoculation, see chapter 5.)

First episodes of genital herpes can be classified in three categories: *primary infection, nonprimary initial infection,* and *recurrent infection.*

Primary infection

The person who experiences a true primary infection has never previously been exposed to any herpes simplex virus. Before infection there is no history of cold sores, there is no history of exposure to cold sores, and no immunity to herpes has ever developed. The absence of specific immunity is crucial, because it allows for easier infection. The body, in its defense against its first attack by herpes, makes antibodies that can neutralize the herpes virus quite effectively. Also, immune cells of the body learn how to target and destroy the virus. As a result, once specific immune cells and antibodies are present, herpes infections are usually much milder.

The first infection is called a primary infection if no previous antibody to either type 1 or type 2 herpes simplex virus is present. It is only possible to know for sure that a person does not have such antibodies by performing a special blood test. Many people with antibodies to either type 1 or type 2 herpes simplex virus have no recollection of cold sores, genital herpes, or any other symptom related to herpes. During a true primary infection, the virus can be inoculated, or transferred, to surrounding areas of skin. Infection may be much more severe because no immunity specific to herpes is yet present. More sores will usually develop during a true primary, especially in women. The person may feel generally sick, usually with a flu-like illness that feels very much like any other viral infection, causing muscle aches and pains and possibly fever and headaches. Primary infection causes a spectrum of disease symptoms, however. For most people, primary infection will actually pass entirely unnoticed or will cause symptoms or signs that are atypical and may be readily misdiagnosed. An atypical primary infection, for example, could produce only a small amount of vaginal discharge, some difficulty with getting urination started, leg pains, headaches, or vaginitis of unknown cause. A woman may only find out she is in the midst of a primary infection when a routine Pap smear comes back showing active cervical herpes. In a recent case I saw, the family physician noted only some mild redness of the cervix.

When genital sores erupt, they usually do so at the site of inoculation, which is usually on the external genitals. Sores generally look like a cluster of small blisters filled with clear or whitish fluid. The classical herpes sore, seen in plate 8a, page 99, is just this: a group of small blisters *(vesicles)* on a red base of inflamed skin.

In many cases, these blisters are never seen, and the first signs of infection are small erosions of the skin called *ulcers*. Ulcers also tend to come in clusters or groups. They may feel like chafing of the skin or some other nonspecific irritation.

In women, herpes sores or lesions are usually on the external genitals, most commonly on the labia (lips) of the vagina. Another common site is the area covered by pubic hair. In men, sores are usually on the foreskin or the shaf.t of the penis or in the pubic area. but the glans (tip of the penis) is also possible territory. More than one of these areas may be affected during primary herpes. Sores may vary in size from very small (one to two millimeters) to very large (one to two centimeters). Sores are usually quite superficial, with the infection on the outermost layer of the skin. During a symptomatic primary infection, the skin often becomes raw, painful, and itchy. There may be a lot of inflammation at this time, because the body is attacking the virus. This response is healthy but may lead to quite a bit of distress. If sores are present around the urethral meatus-the spot where urine exits-urination may be quite uncomfortable. There may be *external dysuria:* a stinging sensation when urine contacts the sores. Some people feel that they have trouble getting the urine stream started. Sores may also appear on the thighs, on the buttocks, or around the anus. There may also be sores in other areas, such as the mouth. If oral contact occurred with the same sores that infected your genitals, a mouth infection may result. Rare sites of infection are the fingers, the breasts, and the eyes.

Often the lymph nodes are swollen in the *inguinal,* or groin, region. This means that the immune system is fighting off the virus. Lymph nodes are those "glands" that the doctor often feels for in the neck when you have a cold. Similar glands are present throughout the body. Those in the groin (see figure 5) are the areas of lymph drainage from the genital area. With genital infection, the groin lymph nodes may become swollen and tender to the touch, since the lymph system is an important component of the body's immune system.

The cervix (the mouth of the womb) is infected about 80 to 90 percent of the time during primary infection. Except for vaginal discharge, cervical infection causes little in the way of symptoms. Occasionally, herpes sores can be seen on the cervix. During primary infection, there is usually some herpes virus on the cervix, even when sores are not present. Infection of the cervix with herpes may cause a runny vaginal discharge. Vaginal discharge could also be caused by another infection going on at the same time, such as trichomoniasis, yeast, or bacterial vaginosis. It is also important to remember that vaginal discharge may be perfectly normal. In fact, whether or not there is discharge, a physician or a specially trained paramedical person must examine you for other treatable infections that may have been transmitted at the same time as herpes.

So, as you can see, primary herpes infections may cause anything from no symptoms to painful sores, sore throat, headache, and muscle pains, either alone or in combination. Symptoms will usually disappear within two to three weeks. The ulcer-like sores eventually scab over and the dry crusts fall off. This marks the end of the primary infection. Occasionally people find that they don't feel quite right for several weeks after their primary infection. There is no good explanation for this feeling.

Nonprimary initial infection

Not all first episodes of herpes are primaries, however. If a person having his or her first clinical experience with the virus is found to have blood test evidence of a previous exposure to type 1 herpes simplex virus, the episode is classified as a nonprimary initial infection. This person has an "immune memory" as a result of previous infection with herpes simplex type 1. More than 50 percent of people have some antibodies to type 1 herpes simplex virus, usually because they were exposed to someone's cold sores in childhood or because of a primary genital infection that gave no symptoms. So, in fact, the first clinical episode of genital herpes is usually not a true primary infection. Strengthening of the body's immune system by previous exposure makes non primary initial herpes very different from primary herpes. The antibodies and lymphocytes have already learned about type 1 herpes and are ready to be quickly activated when triggered by the presence of type 2 herpes. When infection occurs, the body combats the disease effectively and rapidly. The symptoms are essentially the same as for recurrent herpes. Recent studies suggest prove that type 1 herpes antibody partially protects against herpes type 2 infection, acting as a partial "vaccine." Over time, a person with preexisting immunity to herpes type 1 is theoretically less likely to pick up an infection with herpes type 2. However, previous type 1 antibody is clearly not totally protective against herpes type 2, since it is well known that people can acquire type 2 genital herpes after a lifelong history of type 1 (e.g., cold sores). In some studies, people with previous herpes simplex virus type 1 antibodies were almost three times less likely to pick up type 2 from an infected

32

partner over time compared with people who had no previous type 1 herpes exposure. Even if a vaccine were to be only partially protective, though, it could still help, in theory, by raising the threshold of infection. Under such circumstances, it might require more virus, better inoculation, and better transmission circumstances for the body to take the new infection because of its underlying partial immunity. The partial immunity provided by type 1 antibody could thus provide a significant benefit by reducing the overall risk of acquiring type 2. This protection forms the basis of the studies of herpes vaccines currently under way; it has been the hope that vaccines may also provide significant clinical protection against infection. Results so far show that one of the vaccine candidates under study is not effective. Further studies continue with other candidate vaccines.

Recurrent infection

Like the typical non primary first episode, recurrent herpes is usually much milder than primary infection-again because of preexisting immunity to herpes. Like the symptoms of a primary, the symptoms of recurrent herpes are the result of herpes infections of epithelial (skin) cells. However, recurrent infection results when virus travels back down the nerve pathway-often the same nerve fiber the virus originally traveled up on its way to causing latent infection of the ganglion (see figure 4) or a nerve branch from a close-by portion of the ganglion. When a recurrence takes place, however, the immune system is ready to deal with it.

Although the terms may be a bit confusing, we now know that many first episodes of genital herpes are actually recurrences. Even though it is the first clinically noticeable event, a special type-specific blood test (the Western blot) may show that a person is already immune to type 2 herpes simplex virus. This person may have had a primary or non-primary first episode in the past that went totally unnoticed (asymptomatic). Where a first episode is shown by this blood test to be recurrent, transmission may have taken place months or even years before the symptoms were noticed.

Of course, the vast majority of recurrent herpes infections are those that follow the first episode. We have learned, though, that the first episode may be a *primary* infection, a *non-primary* infection, or even a *recurrent* infection that was not previously recognized.

People with recurrent herpes are often troubled very little by physical ailments during recurrences. There are usually few sores. The sores, which may be single or multiple, tend to come in clusters, often grouped together on a small, reddened, inflamed base of skin. Recurrences of herpes go through a series of relatively pre-dictable stages, all of which are described in detail in the next section of this chapter. Unlike primary infection, the recurrent herpes sequence usually takes just a few days from start to finish-an average of six days for men and five days for women. Compared with primary infection, recurrent lesions have less virus in them and are much less uncomfortable. Itchiness is very common. Recurrent sores are often tender to the touch, but they may not hurt a great deal if left alone. If, however, the sores are in a place where they are touched by urine or rubbed, pain may be more prominent. The general feeling of sickness that is usually present in the case of primary infection is now usually absent. Sores are in the same places as in primary herpes, except that the internal genitals and the cervix are much less often affected than in primary infection.

As with primary herpes, the symptoms of recurrent herpes depend on the area affected. Generally, one small area of one of the sites pictured in figure 6 is affected during one recurrence. Some people find that each recurrence is at precisely the same site. Others find that the site varies slightly each time. A sore may hurt when it occurs in one site but itch in another. Different recurrences may be of widely different severity, even in the same spot in the same person.

It is important to reiterate the wide range of severity here. Active recurrent herpes may be obvious when it comes in clusters of little blisters. But genital herpes may never be more severe than one very small sore on the labia or foreskin, around the anus, or on the thigh. It may be the size of a pencil eraser or as small as the sharpened lead point. The sore or chafing may never be painful at all and may not even itch. Herpes is variable and sometimes very atypical; it may hurt over here but itch over there. Assume that any break in the skin in an area depicted in figure 6 is herpes unless you know otherwise. Using a mirror, rub a wet finger lightly over the areas, looking for tender or red or swollen spots that might be active herpes. Get to know your herpes and anything else that is unusual on your genitals. You need to know if you're having a herpes outbreak when you're planning to have sex. If, much of the time, you have only minor skin problems or discomfort that only rarely turns into a classical herpes sore, then there could well be some other explanation for your sensations or skin breaks. For example, you might have a bacterial or yeast vaginal infection or you might be unsure about what is a sore and what is not. On the other hand, being too cavalier about genital discomfort is not good either. People commonly confuse herpes with other things, especially before they get to know their herpes. Herpes is often misidentified as a spider bite, especially on a leg or buttock or in an area remote from the genitals (see plate 9, page 100); a yeast infection (see plate 10, page 100); a hemorrhoid; pimples (on the buttocks, labia, etc.); shingles; water blisters; or cuts, slits, or chafing of the lips of the vagina caused by friction or soreness from vigorous contact.

The appearance and sequence of herpes sores are discussed in the coming pages. (For illustrations, refer to plates on pages 98 and 99.) The spectrum of variable severity must be kept in mind. The phases may all occur in the obvious sequence, or some phases may be skipped. They may last a week or an hour. Rarely, a person may need a hospital bed to recover from herpes. Someone in this situation will usually know the diagnosis! Others will never notice anything unusual. You can reach a happy medium of awareness of your body without overconcern about unrelated twinges. This happy medium may take a few months to achieve, but it will come. When herpes phases are inactive, virus is generally not on the skin, although exceptions to this occur from time to time in nearly all people with genital herpes. Avoiding transmission is relatively straightforward, although it requires a good understanding of the active phases of infection as well as of asymptomatic viral shedding and the susceptibility of the partner to infection. An active recurrence may never occur, or it may occur once in a lifetime, once in a year, or as often as three to four times a month. Type 2 herpes usually recurs at least a few times in the first year following infection. Although type 1 genital herpes can and does recur, the recurrences are about ten to fifteen times less frequent and are not so predictable.

What are the phases of herpes infections?

It is very important to know the phases, because living virus is very likely to be on the skin during the active phases. The phases of infection can be categorized as asymptomatic, prodrome (warning), early redness, edema, vesicles, wet ulcers, crusts, and healed.

During the *asymptomatic* phase, the virus is generally latent.
Living in the ganglion, herpes is usually not on the skin. If you know what herpes feels and looks like and you've looked and found none, you can be confident that the risk of transmission at that specific time is far lower than during one of the active phases of infection. Herpes is only passed on when it is active on the skin. You can do a great deal to prevent transmission. However, there is a small risk that the virus may be reactivating even though your body does not sense an outbreak. Overall, asymptomatic shedding seems to occur on about 1 to 4 percent of days, depending on the patient population and the study. Safer sex consistently practiced during asymptomatic periods is the best way to reduce transmission risks. Suppressive, twice-daily antiviral medication substantially (but not completely) reduces the frequency of asymptomatic shedding. (These issues are discussed again at some length in subsequent chapters.)

Most (but not all) people with recurrences of herpes have a *prodrome,* or warning, that signifies that the virus has been reactivated and is on its way to the skin. As the virus activates, the nerve may react and symptoms may develop. The warning is different for different people. Recurrences often begin with some sensation or warning sign that something is wrong-for example, a pain in the leg or tingling or itching in one area of the genitals. Warning signs, if present, may occur for a few minutes or a few days. If there is a warning sign, it typically develops at the site of the future sore for a few hours before the outbreak begins. It may be a sensation such as localized burning, itching, tingling, or vague discomfort. The most common prodromal symptom is itching at the site before the lesions appear. Sometimes, though, warnings are not directly at the lesion site. Remember that nerves branch and that the virus reactivates very close to the body's central nervous system. Even though effectively eliminated by the immune system, herpes can irritate nerves at the ganglion or nerve site, rather than the skin site. For example, some people with herpes feel leg pains or buttock pains or sensations of burning on the side of the leg or bottom of one foot. Others develop a headache or a feeling like having a cold or the flu. Some people become emotionally irritable or down just before an outbreak. It may be something you've never noticed. It is useful to think about and identify your prodromal phase, if possible, because the prodromal phase tells you that the active sequence has started. At this time about 20 to 25 percent of people begin to have virus present on the skin. Skin contact with genital areas or other areas where you usually get sores should stop until the recurrence is completely over. It is very common for this phase to come and go without other phases following. After it is over, many people realize that they have had a warning, in the form of a vague sensation, below the level of consciousness, that something was amiss. Once a sore is there, there is the recognition, "Oh yeah, I felt that coming all day." Such recognition requires backtracking in your mind. If you have warnings, try to notice them as they occur, because they will help you to learn to recognize the active phase of infection early on. If you have no warnings, then your active phase of infection begins with the development of a lesion.

Next, *early redness* may be detected in a small area of skin (see plate 7a, page 98). It may feel itchy or painful to the touch or just sensitive. At this point, virus is beginning to grow inside the epithelial (skin) cells, and the immune system of antibodies and lymphocytes is being called back to work. The ensuing battle between defenses and virus causes inflammation or redness. Virus is in the skin, so contact with the area where a sore is developing is unwise. Sexual contact with the affected area-even protected sexual contact using safer sex practices-should not take place until the active phases of infection are over.

Soon, a sore begins to develop, beginning as a tiny spot of skin swelling or edema. The degree of swelling varies from one person to another and from one episode to another. Swelling is often so small that I hesitate to even mention this phase. For most people, the amount of skin edema is smaller in size than you might find from a tiny mosquito bite. This phase may be something that can be sensed as a swollen area, or it may be something that is felt by the fingers as one notices a bit of excess tissue at the site of tenderness. Sometimes, these areas of swelling may already have a small sore developing within the small area of swelling. Rarely, swelling from herpes can be very dramatic and result in a big swollen area. Herpes is often missed as the diagnosis in such cases, unless obvious sores are also present.

The next stage is *vesicles* (small blisters) (see plates 7b and Sad, pages 98 and 99). Vesicles are the small blisters filled with clear, whitish, or red (bloody) fluid that form on top of the early red or swollen patch. There may be only one vesicle, a few, or groups of so many that they run together. The tops of these blisters are very thin and come off easily, often oozing a little of the fluid. The fluid is the product of the sick, swollen skin cells that have been attacked by herpes. As the inflammation continues, itchiness and/or pain is often, but not always, present. Virus is virtually always present at this stage, so this is a good time to get a culture diagnosis. However, this stage is commonly skipped, especially in women with labial sores and men with sores under the foreskin, because these wet areas quickly macerate the blister and remove its top, leaving an ulcer underneath. In fact, just touching the vesicles may cause them to break and leak fluid. A vesicle poked with a cotton swab or the tip of your finger will be quite tender, even if it is not bothersome just sitting there. Avoid breaking vesicles on purpose, since there is nothing to be gained by doing this. Vesicles are usually grouped together on a red base of skin. They tend to form most obviously when herpes breaks out in an area where the skin is normally dry-for example, buttock, thigh, pubis, labia majora, or penile shaft.

Following the vesicle stage, lesions evolve into very superficial erosions, or *wet ulcers,* which are really the vesicles with their tops off (see plates 7c, 8e,f, pages 98 and 99). They glisten with wetness and may feel raw and/or tender to the touch. There may be one tiny sore that can be seen only with a magnifying lens, or there may a dozen large, tender ulcers. They may group together to form larger ulcers. Herpes ulcers are superficial; that is, they are right at the skin surface. They are not deep or ragged. They are generally somewhat round and wet. Tender to the touch is the rule, but there are exceptions. Virus is virtually always present at the base of the ulcer. Wet ulcers may look like a small cut or a red, swollen area. Slitlike (straight line) cuts that have absolutely no roundness to them in genital skin folds are often not caused by herpes. If that is all you experience, you should make certain that the sores you are getting are really herpes. Spread away the pubic hair, if necessary, for a good look, and use a magnifying mirror. Touch the sore with a cotton swab or a wet finger again to see if it is tender. This is really the area of the vesicle where the roof of the small blister has been removed. On areas of wet skin (labia minora, under the foreskin of the penis, clitoral hood, perineum, or perianal areas), sores may evolve so quickly that vesicles do not form.

Some people are not familiar or comfortable with identifying these areas as "sores" or "lesions" or "blisters" or "ulcers" because they are so mild in severity. Words like these may conjure up images for you that sound too severe. However, it is important to recognize symptoms, regardless of their severity, because doing so is what allows people who do not feel they have herpes to identify their herpes. Since virus may be present in either mild or painful sores, it is necessary to avoid the natural tendency to leave mild things unnoticed. I am not suggesting an obsession over normalar red spots on the skin. Herpes generally causes a specific sore of some type. The word "chafing" may ring more true for people whose recurrent sores are very mild. Areas of chafing are very superficial and often very small. They may be noticed only by their slight tenderness.

After the ulcer or chafing stage, the fluid in the ulcers begins to dry and some lesions may scab over with a *dry crust,* or scab (see plates 7e and 8h, pages 98 and 99). This phase marks the beginning of healing, and virus begins to disappear. The scab covers the raw ulcer just as a scab grows over a cut. At first the scab may be soft and wet and crumbly (see plates 7d and 8g, pages 98 and 99). If the scab is rubbed away, a wet ulcer remains underneath. As the sore dries, the crust hardens. Underneath, the skin grows anew. This is called re-epithelialization, While the crust is still there, virus may be present. Sexual contact with the area of the sore is still not advisable. The itch or pain may be leaving entirely, or the itch may just begin to worsen at this stage. The size of the lesion generally determines the size of the scab. Some small sores never have a crust stage and seem to melt away from ulcer to nothing. Others always form a dry crust. Scabbing is also very variable and tends to occur mainly on dry skin areas where lesions begin with the vesicle stage.

The sores are *healed* when the crust falls off or the lesion dries without forming a crust, completing the cycle of active infection (see plates 8i,j, page 99). Healing may leave a residual red mark, as a healed cut does. These spots may also be whitish rather than red, or they may in some other way look different from the unaffected skin. The marks may be slightly tender, but the surface is definitely healed with new skin that is smooth and knit back together and feels normal to the touch. The visible mark may last for weeks or for only a few days. Some people never get marks. Virus growth is over; only healing is active at this stage. Safer sexual (protected) contact with this area can now be resumed. In recurrent herpes, the healed phase generally occurs five to ten days after the appearance of the vesicle stage, although the time may be measured in hours or (rarely) in weeks. The "natural history" of a primary herpes outbreak is approximately three weeks. Not every phase occurs in every person. One or several of the phases may be skipped; for example, warnings may occur and no sores develop; ulcers may develop with no warning or blisters; or ulcers may heal with no crust stage. The stages are still important, however. When no symptoms are present and no sores are visible (and you've looked), or when only residual redness is left, the active infection is over and you are in the asymptomatic phase.

What are the trigger factors?

Several studies suggest that latent herpes may reactivate because of trigger factors. These factors are poorly understood, however, and are for the most part unavoidable. The known trigger factors include the menstrual cycle; emotional stress; another illness, especially with fever; sexual intercourse; surgery; injury; sunlight; and certain medications.

Each person's trigger factor is different. For example, while many women get herpes only during a certain part of the menstrual cycle, the trigger day of the cycle varies from woman to woman. One study suggested that more women develop recurrences five to twelve days before the onset of their next menstrual period than at other times. Birth control pills, which stop the normal cycling of hormones, don't seem to diminish recurrences, but careful studies have not been performed.

Emotional stress may be important for some, but for others stress is unrelated to herpes outbreaks. Trying to force away stress in an attempt to rid oneself of herpes may succeed only in making a lot of new stress. Stress has not been proven to cause herpes to recur. In fact, a recent study was unable to show that stress could be correlated with the timing of a new recurrence. Since herpes itself is stressful, how can we be sure which is the chicken and which is the egg? Herpes is a virus infection, not an episode of the jitters. Reactivation of latent infection in the nervous system is a very complex process that remains poorly understood. Easy answers to tough questions-such as how to control triggers-may be misleading and create false hopes. That is not to say that getting rid of stress is not a good idea. About 75 percent of people who have herpes relate their outbreaks to stress and believe that stress control can lead to herpes control. I encourage everyone to take steps to reduce life's stresses. On the other hand, I encourage everyone to avoid feeling that they have failed or are guilty if efforts at stress control do not reduce herpes outbreaks.

Some people say that sexual intercourse leads to sores. This is also a tough one. Often these are healed sores, usually in the residual redness phase, that have a very thin layer of skin over them that tears easily during intercourse. This occurs mainly in people who have very frequent recurrences. They resume sex after healing, only to find a new sore in the morning. This is frustrating indeed, but sex is probably not the trigger. Rather, sex is the innocent victim of unfortunate circumstance. If you feel that sex triggers recurrences, try waiting a few extra days after healing before resuming sexual contact. It may be the abrasion itself. Try slow and gentle sex and lubricants. Make sure that this really is herpes, by returning to your physician with a new sore. Depending on your individual situation, one of the oral antiviral medicines may be useful (see chapter 11).

Surgery and injury are unavoidable. Sunlight, however, can (and should) be avoided by covering affected areas with clothing or sunblocking agents. Dr. S. Spruance of the University of Utah recently presented intriguing data on the use of oral acyclovir in patients who were prone to developing sunlight-triggered cold sores. He treated them effectively, before they developed symptoms at all, by predicting that their cold sores would develop after skiing. He went to the ski slopes to get his volunteers. Oral acyclovir is extremely effective at prevention (see chapter 11), much more effective than when it is used after the beginning of even the earliest symptoms of infection. Dr. Stephen Straus took this in a slightly different direction and showed that sun blockers are effective at reducing the incidence of cold sores triggered by the sun. If we could figure out all the triggers in advance of recurrence onset, sun blockers or antiviral agents could be used intermittently to prevent disease. Thus far, however, the only trigger with this predictability level is sunlight on the lip. Since genital herpes is generally covered by clothing, sunlight is not of practical significance in most people. On the other hand, if you like to tan the areas where you get herpes sores, whether type 1 or type 2, you may find that sunlight is a trigger factor for you. You may wish to stop tanning or use suppressive antiviral medication during the summer. You may also wish to consider the fact that ultraviolet light from the sun is dangerous on its own and is a well-known cause of skin cancer and premature aging.

Before you take any medications, including megavitamins, make sure you need them. Never use cortisone creams or any of the derivatives of cortisone (ask your doctor or pharmacist) to treat herpes. If they must be used for another reason, make sure the reason is a good one. Nothing will help a herpes virus live a long, healthy, active life like cortisone. In fact, any ointment other than specific antiviral medication may prolong the duration of sores. People who have readily identifiable triggers may find themselves in situations where triggers are unavoidable. It is rational to consider prophylaxis with antiviral medication for these periods if you wish. You will find more information about this approach in chapter 11.

If I've had a first episode of herpes, will I have a recurrence? There is no way to predict who will have a recurrence and who will not. Most people will have at least a few. If you have genital herpes simplex virus type 2, you will be more likely to have recurrences than if you have type 1. In fact, type 2 may recur as much as ten to fifteen times as often as type 1 in the genital areas. The reverse is true for facial herpes, where type 1 is far more frequent and recurs much more often. A report by Dr. Lawrence Corey's group at the University of Washington suggests that 84 percent of women and 100 percent of men who have first episodes of type 2 genital herpes have at least one recurrence. For some people, recurrences get milder and less frequent with time, although you should not keep a calendar with the expectation that each recurrence will be shorter than the last. There may be no reduction in the frequency of episodes. The recurrence pattern and severity vary a lot. In fact, if there is one thing you can be sure of, it is that the recurrence pattern will change from time to time. It is this shifting pattern of recurrences that makes the many false cures for herpes seem to work for some people. Such cures turn out to offer no real benefit after rigorous testing. Overall, the average number of recurrences of type 2 genital herpes is about four per year. However, up to 40 percent of people will experience six or more and up to 20 percent of people will experience ten or more symptomatic recurrences in the first year.

Recurrences of herpes can start even as the primary infection heals. Recurrences may overlap, or one may begin as another is ending. They may occur first on the labia and next on the thigh. Episode sites may rotate from one site to another or stay repeatedly in the same place. No treatment during the initial episode has yet been devised that will affect the pattern of future recurrences. Recent studies in animals, however, have suggested that very early treatment with some antiviral medicines may have a long-term benefit. Clinical studies are underway. The reasons for differences in recurrence patterns are not known.

Is it possible to have herpes without any symptoms?

Several studies have shown that antibody directed against type 2 herpes is detected by the Western blot blood test very commonly in people who do not have a history that even suggests genital herpes. Similarly, herpes frequently can be found (if looked for in a research study) in its latent state inside neurons in the sacral ganglia of autopsy cases in which this diagnosis was never suspected and where the person had never reported any symptoms. Furthermore, most people with herpes have not had any contact that they know of with a person with herpes. Similarly, the unknowingly infected sexual partner of someone with a new case of primary genital herpes will usually deny ever having had symptoms of either genital herpes or oral-labial herpes. Even in a private room with a physician listing symptoms, most people will have great difficulty identifying the symptoms of genital herpes until they have understood how mild these sores can be in their recurrent state. As a comparison, the mild mosquito bite that healed a week ago may barely be remembered (if at all) next to the often severe symptoms the primary patient is experiencing. There is often a mistaken expectation that "If the diagnosis is genital herpes in 'my partner with the primary,' then genital herpes in me must look and/or feel the same way." However, genital herpes commonly causes no symptoms at all. In fact, most cases of genital herpes are never recognized unless they are transmitted to someone else, and sometimes not even then. The expectation that a severe infection in one partner will be matched by an infection of equal severity in the other partner is absolutely wrong. Sexually transmitted diseases are most often transmitted from an asymptomatic partner (or sometimes from a partner who does not notice the symptoms) to someone who then may get very severe symptoms. Dr. Anna Wald at the University of Washington recently reported her study of people who tested positive by the Western blot test for type 2 herpes but in whom symptoms of herpes had never been noticed. She found that these people were just as likely to have virus on their genital skin with no symptoms as were people who were already aware of their diagnosis because of sores and symptoms. Sometimes, of course, both partners stay asymptomatic until partners change and a subsequent partner develops more severe symptoms. At this point, patients and couples often become very confused. They ask partners about symptoms and begin to suspect things. Of course, occasionally a partner is lying. But the story of who infected whom can get pretty complicated in a lot of cases. Before you accuse, remember that many people who point fingers at someone for transmitting herpes point in the wrong direction.

The explanation for this confusion is not clear. However, it is easy to see how a mild herpes blister that looks like a pimple or a tiny pinhole might go unnoticed. Even a really severe infection, if localized to the cervix or other internal genital area, may cause no symptoms whatsoever. An infinite number of scenarios to explain asymptomatic transmission can be imagined. For example, a recurrent sore around the anus may cause recurrent rectal itching. This is a symptom that nearly everyone has at one time or another and could easily be passed off as insignificant. Can anyone honestly deny ever having had an itch in the rectum-even one that recurs from time to time?

Does herpes always hurt?

Herpes usually does not hurt much. Severe symptoms are most prominent during the primary infection. Sores that are open and raw are commonly tender or painful to touch. Push a cotton swab on a sore and it will hurt. Urinate on a sore and it will hurt. Itching may be more common than pain during recurrences. Pain is a funny thing. People sense pain differently. Some people with recurrent herpes never feel anything and only know that the herpes is active by looking at the sores. Others are exquisitely aware of the slightest change in their body's chemistry. Regardless, pain is usually not the major problem in coping with recurrent herpes.

On the other hand, patients with strong primary infections may suffer extreme pain for a short time. It may be too painful to urinate, to sit, or to walk. Hospitalization with intravenous antiviral therapy and painkillers maybe required. It can be very frightening to imagine this pain recurring every month for a lifetime. Happily, it does not. If you are reading this during your primary, keep in mind that although herpes may recur, it will never again do what it is doing now. Recurrent herpes is not a recurrence of primary herpes. It is generally much milder. Sores are smaller and less painful and are usually gone after several days.

Can herpes cause other kinds of pain?

Because herpes likes nerves, it may cause irritation there. During reactivation (the prodrome phase) the virus travels down the nerve and may cause pain in other areas where the nerve runs. This pain, called *sacral paresthesia,* is often in the leg or buttocks and usually disappears when the prodrome phase is over. Headache may also be a warning sign. Often during a bad primary infection and rarely with a recurrent infection, the reactivating virus travels up the nerve as well as down, finding its way into the central nervous system to cause *meningitis-an* inflammation of the sac around the brain. This inflammation, if caused by herpes, is not generally harmful. It does not damage the nervous system, although it can be quite distressing, resulting in headache, stiff neck, aversion to bright lights, and fever. It does get better quickly. If meningitis occurs, seek the care of a physician so you can be sure that it is just herpes. (Meningitis may require specific therapy.) An unusual, but not rare, complaint after an active recurrence is *postherpetic neuralgia,* or residual pain in the area involved. The skin may feel painful, prickly, itchy, numb, throbbing, cold, hot, or as if it is drawn too tightly. Postherpetic neuralgia generally fades with time. This syndrome is unfortunately very common following herpes zoster (shingles) infection, especially in people who are over the age of fifty or have severe pain when the rash begins. Note that it *follows* active infection and thus does not represent active viral shedding; it is an inactive phase. Other kinds of discomfort occur in some people after a bout of genital herpes. In such cases, shooting pains or aching in the buttock or down the back of one or both legs persists far beyond what one would expect from a simple reactivation of herpes. Presumably, this pain results from a bit of residual nerve damage near the spinal cord, where herpes established its latent infection. If inflammation occurs there, it may be called *radiculitis*. It is usually best to leave the pain untreated and wait for it to fade. However, the physician should decide with you on the best approach. It is important to tell your physician about the symptoms so that he or she can determine that it is only herpes and nothing more serious. Once that is established, there are various treatment options. Sometimes, patients find that trying to control this discomfort with drugs is worse than the problem itself. The only treatment sure not to have adverse effects is no treatment at all. Antiherpesvirus drugs are not especially effective in this setting, although they may be worth a try. Other drugs used for post-herpetic pain include amitryptyline (Elavil), or other tricyclic antidepressants. Neurologists and pain specialists know how to use these drugs. Whatever you do, though, avoid narcotics for post-herpetic pain, if possible. Narcotic analgesics may be very useful for acute pain of herpes-e.g., during or shortly after primary infection, if absolutely necessary. But post-herpetic pain can last quite a long time in some people, and serious drug addiction may result if narcotics are used. Pain and discomfort are common after herpes zoster (shingles) but, luckily, are relatively rare after herpes simplex infection. Get good medical help with this one if it happens to you.

Can herpes make me sterile?

No, but a number of other sexually transmitted infections-for example, *gonorrhea* and *Chlamydia-can* cause sterility. These infections need to be treated with antibiotics in order to stop them from causing harm. The most common warning signs are (male) urethral or (female) vaginal discharge, painful urination, and a painful lower abdomen. These internal genital infections can cause enough inflammation around the ovaries and tubes in a woman to result in scarring, which makes it difficult for the egg to reach the womb. A culture test and examination for pus cells will generally detect these internal genital infections. Many men and women have no symptoms whatsoever of these infections. The doctor who diagnoses herpes should also test for these infections, especially since they are easy to cure with certain antibiotics. In addition, herpes may be confused with *syphilis* and other diseases, even by the most expert, most widely experienced physician. Only laboratory tests can distinguish the different sexually transmitted infections with 100 percent accuracy. Make sure you undergo these tests at least once, usually during your first episode.

Can herpes make me impotent?

Impotence means that a man is unable to obtain and/or sustain an erection when he feels like doing so. Herpes often has a detrimental effect on feeling like it, especially during the period of anger that commonly occurs after people acquire herpes. Emotions such as anger, depression, and hopelessness about having an "incurable" infection commonly influence sexual urges in men and women with herpes. Usually such changes in urges can be corrected by getting over the fear of talking about herpes with your partner. Changes in sexual urges are normal and common. They should not last for a long time.

Severe primary herpes infections, especially in homosexual men with proctitis (rectal-anal infection), may uncommonly result in physical impotence as a result of nerve inflammation. The inflammation leaves after the acute infection and generally does not recur. There are other more common physical causes for impotence, however, such as diabetes mellitus, certain drugs, and hormonal imbalances. If impotence or loss of sexual desire is sustained, you should seek specific medical attention for the problem.

Are cold sores (fever blisters) also herpes?

Yes, for the most part, fever blisters are caused by herpes simplex. The virus is usually (but not always) type 1. Type 2 herpes of the mouth can also cause cold sores, although type 1 is more efficient than type 2 at causing recurrences on the face. (The converse is true for genital sores: type 2 is more efficient than type 1 at causing recurrences on the genitals.) Sores generally look like genital herpes, but they occur on the lip or the skin near the lip. Mouth herpes-like genital herpes-is most often an external disease. The classic cold sore occurs at the vermilion border of the lipthe point where the thin mucous membrane of the mouth changes abruptly into the skin of the face (see figure 12, page 202). Ulcers in the side of the mouth may be herpes but are usually *aphthous ulcers*, which are not infectious. Cracks in the corners of the mouth are usually not caused by herpes.

True cold sores go through a sequence of active phases similar to the sequence already described. The ganglion for cold sore latency is the *trigeminal ganglion*, located inside the skull. The trigeminal sensory nerve comes from this site and supplies sensation to all parts of the face. This nerve is divided into three branches: the *ophthalmic* branch, which provides sensation to the forehead and eye; the *maxillary* branch, which provides sensation to the cheek and side of the nose; and the *mandibular* branch, which provides sensation to the mouth and chin. The mouth is the most common site of herpes recurrences. Virus traveling to the mouth must travel down the mandibular branch of the trigeminal nerve. Regardless of where herpes is inoculated, it will occur along very well defined nerve pathways, following nerve fibers much like a train staying on its track. The track is chosen back at the ganglion level.

Sounds like genital herpes is a bit like a cold sore of the genitals? That's correct. A person with mouth herpes can give a sexual partner genital herpes by having oral-to-genital contact while oral infection is active. The nature of herpes sores and the sites affected depend largely on what gets inoculated where. The primary inoculation site determines where the first lesions will form and which ganglion will subsequently be infected (back at the train station). Recurrence sites, however, are determined by the skin site where the specific nerve fiber (or train track) ends. Usually, the sites of primary inoculation and subsequent recurrence are very closely related, because one nerve ganglion tends to supply sensation to a small, defined area. Occasionally, the two sites may seem to be far apart (e.g., genital herpes recurring on the buttocks), simply because of the nature of nerve branching. The herpes virus does not travel between ganglia, however, so a person with cold sores need not worry that sores will suddenly appear on his or her genitals. If a person gets sores in two sites supplied by two different ganglia, he or she must have been inoculated at both sites. If your cold sores contact the skin of another person during an active phase, the person will become infected and subsequently establish latent infection at the site where the virus was inoculated.

Can J have received my infection months or even years before my first symptoms?

Yes. Although primary genital herpes is usually quite uncomfortable, it often occurs without any symptoms. Unusual symptoms not readily recognized as herpes are also possible. Remember that herpes infections form a spectrum from no symptoms to severe symptoms. Initial infection may pass unnoticed, and recurrent herpes with symptoms may begin later.

A true primary infection, however, with pain, numerous lesions, fever, etc., is unlikely to have been caused by an infection a long time before. The incubation period for primary herpes is between two and thirty days in general. If your first outbreak is mild, it could actually be a recurrent infection-the first recurrence after an asymptomatic primary infection that took place weeks, months, or even years before. In this case, the incubation period is more difficult to pinpoint. If a Western blot test (see chapter 4) is performed early in the first episode, it can identify the episode as either a true primary, a nonprimary initial episode (previous type 1 herpes exposure), or recurrent herpes (previous type 2 herpes exposure). In one study, seventeen of twenty-four people experiencing first episodes of genital herpes were found to have pre-existing antibodies to herpes simplex type 2 and thus were not having true primaries. Most people with pre-existing immunity to herpes at the time of the first clinical episode are experiencing a recurrence after a primary infection that passed unnoticed at some time in the past. Some may be experiencing their first symptoms of a process that began with transmission at a much earlier date. Remember that an incubation period is identifiable only if it is clear that a true primary infection is taking place or if the Western blot blood test proves this fact. By definition, a person with a true primary is seronegative (blood test for herpes completely negative) at the onset of symptoms because that person has not yet had time to raise antibodies against the virus. Separation of a true primary from a nonprimary first episode or recurrence can be very difficult without this blood test

I often have prodromal symptoms but no sores. What does that mean?

Warning signs without sores probably means reactivation. Most people who have warning symptoms with sores will also have them without sores. The virus has reactivated and may have traveled to the skin, but the body has somehow stopped the infection before it could cause sores. This is very common. In Vancouver, we showed several years ago that about 20 percent of all prodromes will abort without further lesion development, even in the absence of any treatment.

During the prodrome, however, herpes should be considered to be active for a short time. Examine yourself after the warning is over. Sometimes people who believe they do not get sores after the prodrome are not looking closely enough. People with herpes may want to use a mirror, preferably with a well-magnified side, for self-examination. Use a flashlight or another light source that can be brought near to the skin. Remember that sores may vary, may be very small, and may not hurt much. If no signs of herpes occur on the skin, wait a couple of days and resume normal skin contact. If sores develop, follow the phases and wait until the herpes is inactive. It may turn out that many of these *false prodromes* are just that-false. They may be only fleeting neuralgia from the last episode.

False prodromes also occur in some people taking regular oral antiviral medication for prevention of recurrences. Perhaps the recurrent episode begins in the nerve and cycles on but is then aborted before the development of a visible lesion. The significance of these short episodes is unknown. For now, treat them as if they were short recurrences, whether they occur on treatment or off.

Can herpes cause headaches?

Yes, indeed, there is a herpes headache. Headache is very common during a true genital herpes primary infection. Primary her-

51

pes is commonly complicated by meningitis, and meningitis headaches are generally quite severe. This is rarely the case in recurrent herpes. Headache may also be associated with other symptoms, such as stiff neck, nausea, and pain from bright light and loud noises. If it occurs during primary herpes, your doctor may choose to perform a lumbar puncture (needle in the low back) so that a sample of spinal fluid can be examined. This is a very safe procedure and generally causes about the same amount of discomfort as a blood test. Some people get a headache from the lumbar puncture test. The test is necessary only where meningitis is considered significant. It is important in some cases to make sure that other causes of meningitis are not present. Herpes meningitis is generally benign; that is, it gets better on its own without treatment and generally does not recur. However, herpes meningitis is often treated with antiviral medications. This is a decision for you and the doctor to make when the diagnosis is considered.

Alternatively, headache may be the symptom of a prodrome.
Generally, this headache is mild and has no known cause. In fact, most headaches have no known cause. Being sick with anything can cause a headache. Fever can bring on a headache. Tension from herpes or anything else can bring on a headache. If headaches are very severe, whether you feel they are related to herpes or not, you should discuss the problem with your doctor. Herpes does not generally cause chronic headache.

What other symptoms can herpes cause?

Genital herpes is still a poorly understood disease in many ways. We do not know how many people have it or how many know they have it. We do not know everything it can do. We probably know only some of the symptoms.

The symptoms of herpes are usually related to the sores. If the sores are near the urethra, it may hurt to urinate. If they are on the buttocks, it may hurt to sit. Sometimes, however, herpes causes invisible problems. Some people have recurring leg pain. The pain usually radiates down the back of one leg. It may occur in the thigh. Occasionally, this pain may occur without any sores, like a false prodrome. If it is *episodic* (comes and goes) and is usually followed by sores on the skin, then it is likely a prodrome and should be considered a sign of active herpes. If it is *chronic* (always there or takes weeks to go away), chances are it is not related to herpes. With chronic pain, other causes must be ruled out by a physician. In some cases, pain from herpes can be persistent, long after the virus itself has. stopped activity on the skin. Persistent pain after herpes simplex or herpes zoster infection is called *postherpetic neuralgia.* The discomfort of postherpetic neuralgia is usually very similar to the kinds of discomfort experienced during the primary infection; possible symptoms include deep buttock aching, shooting pains down the leg, and numbness in the feet.

During primary infection, any number of unusual things may occur. Primary herpes affects the whole body. Meningitis, as previously described, is common during primary herpes. Very rarely, severe consequences have resulted from herpes, such as severe paralysis from a complication called *transverse myelitis.* Lasting paralysis of muscles from genital herpes is extremely rare, but short-term mild paralysis is not rare during severe primary infection. We have recently seen a patient whose only symptoms during primary genital herpes were leg and bladder weakness with retention of some urine. Absolutely no genital or non genital lesions were ever seen on this patient. The paralysis was minor and she recovered promptly. Temporary difficulties with urination and weakness in some muscles sometimes occur during primary infection, whether or not sores are present. In fact, minor urinary abnormalities are probably much more common than has been recognized. Where these complications occur, function almost always reverts back to normal after a few weeks.

Occasionally a patient with herpes gets abdominal (stomach) pains from primary herpes. I have been told about patients who have actually undergone surgery for appendicitis only to find out they have primary genital herpes. Gonorrhea and Chlamydia are much more likely causes of abdominal pain than herpes is and are very common causes of *pelvic inflammatory disease* (PID), which often causes lower abdominal pain and may result in sterility. These infections need to be treated by a trained person who must look for them and take a culture in order to identify them.

A curious disease called *erythema multiiorme* causes a skin rash with target lesions that look like rings of redness with central color changes (see plate 11, page 100). In addition, the mucous membranes of the mouth, eyes (conjunctiva), or genitals may ulcerate and become painful and raw. Unlike the ulcers of active herpes phases, these ulcers are not infectious. They are generally thought to be a hyperimmune reaction. The body's immune system not only has responded but has overresponded in its efforts to stop the active virus infection during that episode. A few normal cells are damaged by the immune reaction as well, resulting in a rash and ulcers, One of the many causes of erythema multiforme is herpes simplex. Other typical causes include use of certain medications, such as sulfa-containing antibiotics and nonsteroidal anti-inflammatory drugs (NSAIDs) such as aspirin and ibuprofen. Anyone individual with herpes is very unlikely to develop this disease, as is anyone individual who takes NSAIDs or sulfa drugs. Treatment is sometimes simple and sometimes difficult. Cortisone may be called for and is usually taken by mouth rather than as a cream. The disease may relapse. It needs medical attention. Treatment with antiviral medication is often advisable, and suppression may be indicated in some patients. Discuss treatment with your physician.

Now that I have herpes, am I especially prone to other infections? Not long ago, doctors were taught that secondary infection of the skin-for example, staph infection or *impetigo-was* a common complication of herpes. This is now known to be false. More than 99 percent of people with herpes have no other infection. Rarely, staph or strep (two common and easily treated bacteria) invade the skin at the site broken by a herpes sore. Where secondary infection occurs, it results in a clinically distinct syndrome different from the usual course of herpes. Patients with these rare complications may develop a syndrome called *cellulitis* (a very uncommon secondary bacterial infection resulting from herpes). A picture of a patient with cellulitis of the groin is shown in plate 12, page 101. The cellulitis rash is quite different from the usual herpes sores. It has a deep red appearance and is often associated with tenderness and fever. Patients with such problems need urgent medical attention and are usually treated with antibiotics in order to clear the secondary bacterial infection. Another type of secondary infection results in each separate vesicle becoming infected and filled with pus (a sticky and thick substance containing inflammatory cells) and often causes an otherwise typical outbreak to persist longer and be more red than usual. Again, antibiotics are indicated.

Because you have acquired one sexually transmitted disease, there is a small statistical risk that you have acquired another at the same time. This possibility does not have to do with your susceptibility but only with your statistical chances of having caught something else. The other common sexually transmitted infections (gonorrhea, Chlamydia, Trichomonas) and those easily confused with herpes because of the way they look (syphilis, chancroid, shingles) should be ruled out. This is discussed in detail in chapter 4.

People whose immunity is compromised by something unrelated to herpes-for example, cancer, lymphoma, leukemia, transplantation, or acquired immune deficiency syndrome (AIDS)-may get herpes simplex infections that do not heal readily, because their immunity problems make them more susceptible to problematic herpes.

Recent studies have shown that there is one correlation between herpes and human immunodeficiency virus (HIV). Specifically, people with herpes (as well as virtually any other genital ulcer disease) are statistically more likely to have acquired human immunodeficiency virus infection than are people who do not have any genital ulcer disease. There are two possible explanations. First, both infections are sexually transmitted, so it is not surprising that they may be found together. Second, the immune cells that fight off infection with any genital ulcer disease are highly concentrated at the site of a sore or genital ulcer. In the base of the ulcer, fighter cells called "helper" lymphocytes or CD4+ cells work to protect the body from further invasion by whichever infection is causing the genital ulcer. Such cells are the main target cells for attack by the human immunodeficiency virus. So, if HIV is pre-

sent during sexual contact and if the cells containing this virus find a genital ulcer conveniently available, then HIV can find ready entry into its prime target cell. In fact, virtually all diseases that lead to genital ulcers result in the same situation-an easy target. Thus, even though there is some association of these two viruses, one does not cause the other. To get *HN,* you have to be exposed to HIV If, when you are exposed to *HN,* you have an unhealed genital ulcer, your risk of actually acquiring HIV on that occasion goes up somewhat. But having herpes alone does not cause HIV infection. In fact, people who are careful about avoiding herpes transmission do not have sexual contact during the active ulcer stage anyway.

Herpes infection might actually lessen the risk of HIV infection in many people; people who acquire herpes tend to reduce their exposure risk to HIV by reducing their numbers of sexual partners and adopting safer sexual practices. Dr. Suzanne Kroon of Denmark has called this change in lifestyle, "increasing the quality control [of partners]." It is one of the real benefits of having genital herpes, and it could conceivably save your life. People with herpes who elect to ignore these risk factors do run the risk of acquiring HIV and, if exposed, are approximately twice as susceptible to actually becoming infected compared with people who do not have recurrent genital sores.

Genital Herpes: The Diagnosis

How is the diagnosis made?

In some situations, genital herpes may be a simple diagnosis for the general practitioner. In others, it may elude the specialist. When symptoms and signs of herpes are "classical"-that is, when exposure is known to have taken place and painful clustered vesicles (blisters) or ulcers have developed on a red, inflamed base-the clinical diagnosis is clear-cut. Recurrences make herpes even more likely. Then, the virus itself is detected by a culture test from one of the sores, confirming the diagnosis. In order to make sure that no other diseases accompany herpes, tests for syphilis, gonorrhea, Chlamydia, Trichomonas, HIV, and yeast are also performed.

On the other hand, some people with genital herpes have mild intermittent symptoms. The only sore may be a single pinpoint ulcer on the labia that lasts for a few days, occurs every six months, and does not hurt at all. The diagnosis may not even occur to the patient or the physician. A virus culture test to detect herpes in the sore should be performed during an active phase of infection. If the test is positive, herpes is likely to be the cause of the sore. A positive culture for herpes simplex virus from the skin means that you have herpes. The virus culture is so reliable, it is called the gold standard for this infection.

If the test is negative, however, herpes mayor may not be the cause of the problem. Consider the phases of herpes (discussed in chapter 3). Was the test obtained during an active period? If not, it can be expected to be negative, even if herpes is the problem. Even if the period was an active one, quite often herpes virus is not recoverable. How was the test obtained? Was the doctor's office far away from the laboratory? If so, the virus may not have survived the trip. How experienced is the laboratory? This varies. Some laboratories save money by dividing up clinical samples into extremely small samples, so that they can actually perform 96 different viral culture tests on the surface of one plastic plate. Such costsavers will reduce the sensitivity of the test. Most quality laboratories are certified by the College of American Pathologists (CAP) or whatever governing body for accreditation is applicable in your area. Even under ideal circumstances, virus recovery in the laboratory after only one try is not always possible.

If you suspect herpes and your doctor agrees, your best bet is to return again for virus culture at the first sign of recurrence. The earlier the specimen is obtained, the better the chance of an accurate test. In my experience, two visits will suffice, if the visits are early. If herpes is suspected and cultures are negative, it is probably best to try to obtain a Western blot (blood) test. This test is described later in this chapter.

I have been exposed to someone who has herpes. Should I go to my doctor now for a test?

This is an increasingly common question. It is also a difficult problem. If you have been exposed to someone with herpes, the person's herpes may have been active or inactive.

If your partner's herpes was in an inactive stage, your risk is very low. If no symptoms develop, you do not need to do anything. Nothing will almost certainly be what continues to happen unless you become exposed, in the future, to an active infection.

If your partner's infection was in an active stage, you may have come into contact with the virus. Whether or not you will develop herpes depends on several factors.

Was there virus present? The active stages are a good guess for when exposure risk is high, but often sores contain no living virus. If sores were active, you may have been infected, but not necessarily so.

The number of virus particles (inoculum) is important. If the inoculum that made contact was very high, then infection is more likely. If virus was present in very small amounts, infection is less likely.

Where did inoculation take place? Was this contact through thin skin-for instance, on the genitals? Were there cuts on the skin? Was contact prolonged? Did a long time elapse before washing the area? Are you female? (Women have about three to four times more risk of being infected than men.) All of these things might increase the chance for any virus to transfer from one person to another.

Several other "host factors" also playa role. If you already have antibody to type 1 herpes simplex virus (more than half of North Americans have this without knowing it), a higher dose of herpes simplex virus type 2 is probably required to result in infection. If you already have herpes simplex virus type 2 (about 20 percent of North American people have this antibody without knowing it), you may not really even be at any substantial risk of catching genital herpes at all, since you already have it. The immune system may also be an important factor in some ways we do not understand.

Whether or not you develop symptoms of herpes will determine the type of diagnostic test you require. If no symptoms are present, only the Western blot test can be used to diagnose genital herpes. This is one occasion when you need to be very careful about what information the doctor has when the diagnosis is made or excluded. It might be a good idea to show your doctor this chapter to make sure that you are both talking about the same issues. By performing a history and physical examination and cultures for virus, the doctor can rule out problems other than genital herpes. If you have symptoms, this examination may tell you what you do have. Examination and culture alone, however, cannot exclude what you do not have. In other words, if you do not have an active sore at the time you are examined, the doctor cannot correctly conclude, on this basis, that you do not have genital herpes. The same is true of a partner. If a viral culture test for herpes comes up positive, of course, that does correctly diagnose herpes. A negative culture test, though, does not exclude the diagnosis. Why? Because herpes is recurrent, with a lot of inactive and unpredictable episodic time between relapses. The examination and viral culture test would come up negative most of the time even in a person who has herpes, because the virus is inactive most of the time. If symptoms develop-e.g. vaginal discharge, sores, unexplained tenderness of the genitals, redness, pimples, or swollen lymph nodes-then go to the doctor without delay. If there is no other obvious cause for the symptoms, and exposure to herpes is likely, inform the doctor and ask for a herpes culture. Go early, when symptoms are present. Waiting it out does not help. Herpes will go away on its own, only to probably return again. If you want to know (and it is your responsibility to know), go to the doctor when symptoms first appear.

The most advanced blood test for herpes, currently available in a few centers, is the *Western blot test.* If a visible sore is present, this test is unnecessary, since the virus culture test not only is the gold standard but is also cheaper and is often a better, more direct means of detecting the presence of virus. The blood test is described later in this chapter. The blood test to rule out herpes after a possible exposure may be especially useful, since sores often do not develop and people still want to know if they were exposed. The blood test cannot tell you where you were exposed, but it can be used to determine if type 2 herpes simplex virus infection is present. The type-specific antibody test must be performed at least twelve weeks after a possible exposure in order to be reasonably sure that a negative result truly means that you probably have not acquired herpes. In the best hands, this test is very accurate, but no test is 100 percent sensitive. Occasionally, even the best test misses the mark. In some people, it takes several weeks to convert to a positive. The type-specific test is just coming into its own, however. The test is difficult to get. It is the best test for this situation, currently, but different labs do things differently. Before having the test done at a laboratory, be sure that the test:

1. is type-specific by testing at least for *glycoprotein G-2* (gG-2) by Western blot or some other proven method and,

2. is well controlled. What is the lab's sensitivity rate? (In other

words, how often does this lab come up with a negative test that is falsely negative (incorrect)?) The best Western blot tests are close to 99 percent accurate. Ask your health care provider about this.

You might consider taking a course of one of the oral antiviral agents against herpes because of virus exposure before developing symptoms (see chapter 11) if: 1.) you feel your exposure to an active herpes sore was fairly certain, 2.) you feel that you may be susceptible to getting herpes (do not already have the same type of herpes as your partner), and 3.) your exposure happened within the past few days (preferably fewer than three days).

How is the diagnosis proven?

The best way to prove that herpes is present, regardless of how sure it looks, is with a test that shows herpes simplex virus to be present in a sore. The most sensitive test (the most likely to show positive when it is herpes) is a culture test. Since virus lives inside cells, a few of the cells from a sore must be taken and sent for culture. A wet cotton or Dacron swab is rolled into a sore, put into a special salt solution, and sent to the laboratory.

At the lab, some of the fluid is removed and placed onto healthy human cells that are kept growing in tubes. The cells are called a tissue culture. Once virus is placed onto the tissue culture, it is called a virus culture. The laboratory technician keeps the cells growing at body temperature in an incubator and, during the next several days, removes the culture from the incubator and places it under the microscope. If the cells remain healthy, the culture is negative. If the cells become sick from herpes, they will round up and group themselves together. This change in appearance is called the *cytopathic effect* (ePE). An area of herpes infection of cells called *fibroblasts* is shown in figure 8. Note the long, pointed, wispy appearance of the normal cells, on the upper left, compared to the sick-looking swollen cells where the virus is growing, to the left of the bracket.

Once the ePE has occurred, the technician puts a small number of cells from the tube onto a slide and adds a herpes simplex antibody to the slide. The antibody is usually attached to a chemical that fluoresces (emits light) under ultraviolet (UV) light. If the cells fluoresce, the changes in the cells must have been caused by herpes simplex. A positive fluorescence test is shown in plate 4, page 97. The bright areas on the cells are fluorescing because herpes antibody is stuck to the virus on the cell. Note the apple green rim containing the fluorescent dye linked to the antibody.

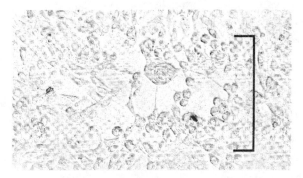

Figure 8: *Microscopic appearance of cells affected by herpes simplex virus. Normal cells in culture are altered by the infection taking place in the test tube. Cells are swollen and fused. This is called the cytopathic effect (or CPE) and is suggestive of herpes simplex infection.*

Several other methods of diagnosis may also be used. If fluid is present-e.g., inside a vesicle-the virus may be seen under an electron microscope, a very powerful (and very expensive) piece of equipment about the size of a small car. An experienced and capable technician must operate the machine. Identification of herpes-like particles is truly an art (see figure 3, page 32). Interpretation may be very difficult and, unfortunately, occasionally misleading. All herpes viruses look the same under the electron microscope. Nobody can say, just from this test, if the virus is type 1 or type 2 or even if it is shingles. Furthermore, even though the machine is powerful, it is not sensitive. One must have a lot of virus in a very carefully collected specimen in order to obtain a positive electron microscope test. One must further have great faith in the talents of the technician.

The fluorescent antibody technique described above for cells in culture can also be performed directly on clinical specimens, or a smear from the sore can be put onto a microscope slide and examined directly (a Pap smear). If herpes causes giant cells to form, the giant cells can be seen in the microscope directly. Special stains can be done on the slide, which is then called a *Tzanck smear*.

The smears, the fluorescence, and the electron microscopy tests are quick tests. Others are being developed, as well. In general, compared to culture tests these quick answer tests sacrifice accuracy for speed or convenience. A herpes diagnostic kit called Herpchek, made by Dupont, is very easy for labs to use and is just as sensitive as the culture test. This test is very accurate, but it does not "type" the virus (i.e. determine if it is herpes simplex virus type 1 or type 2). It is called an *enzyme immunoassay* (EIA). EIA is a method of testing either blood or a swab for herpes. The method may be adequate for a swab test but not yet for a type-specific blood test.

Many laboratories now use an extremely sensitive test called the *polymerase chain reaction test* (PCR). PCR is far more sensitive than a culture test and can detect even a few molecules of herpes DNA on the skin. It is currently three to four times as expensive as a culture test and about twice the expense of a Western blot.

Which test to do depends on the situation. Sometimes it is necessary to do more than one type of test. Each of these methods provides direct evidence of herpes infection and, if positive, proves that herpes is present. A negative result on one specific virus test does not prove that herpes is not present. If there is a negative finding, the Western blot test described below is the best way to go.

Is there a blood test for herpes?

Can I take a blood test to accurately determine the presence of herpes? Yes. In fact, this test has markedly improved physicians' ability to properly counsel both patients and their partners. Herpes blood tests measure the body's immune response against the virus. Without infection, there is no specific reaction to the virus. In contrast, shortly after a true viral infection, the body responds to fight the infection. The herpes blood test measures that response by measuring the body's antibody to herpes. All herpes antibody tests do essentially the same thing. They do not directly measure virus. They measure, instead, the body's reaction to the virus. To look directly for virus, one must test a sore containing virus and grow the virus in the laboratory. This has the advantage of determining not only the virus and its type but also what the sores look like and whether or not they contain virus. Because of its dependence on the active sore, however, the virus culture test also has some key disadvantages. To get a positive test from a culture, a person with herpes must have symptoms. Without symptoms, there is nothing to test. Furthermore, the sore must be tested at just the right moment. If it is too early, there may not be an adequate quantity of infected cells. If it is too late in the course of a recurrence, the virus may have already been killed by the body's defenses.

An accurate blood test for herpes antibody has been needed for a long time. An accurate blood test, such as the Western blot, could be used to help diagnose herpes in people who do not even get sores and in people who get them only rarely. People who might want such a test would include the partner who is asymptomatic but may have been the source of herpes. Other blood test candidates would be the person with only one past episode whose culture was lost on the way to the lab, people who think they have been exposed to herpes but are not sure, and couples who want to give up safer sex precautions. If you have no trouble getting a viral test directly from a sore during an active phase, then that is the preferred approach. But if this presents difficulty for any reason, the Western blot is preferred.

Most commercial herpes antibody (blood) tests are not typespecific. All they can tell you is that you have *herpes* of some sort. (positive results on these tests are common since 50 to 80 percent of people over twenty have antibodies to the herpes simplex virus.) Unfortunately, many of the commercial blood tests advertised as *type-specific* widely available to doctors are not very accurate at doing what they claim to do-determining whether you have type 1 or type 2 herpes. Even though they may be based on type-specific laboratory markers, most of them correlate only poorly to the actual clinical situation. These tests (which include enzyme immunoassays [EIA], complement fixation tests, and tests for immunoglobulin M [IgM]) are simply not yet sufficiently accurate for a proper diagnosis of genital herpes. This will probably change in the future. These tests *are* still clinically useful at present, however, in that they can be used to detect antibodies to herpes in the blood and, therefore, determine whether a first episode of genital herpes-already diagnosed by viral culture and typingis a true primary or a nonprimary.

Accurate type-specific antibody tests that have recently been developed test directly for the body's reaction (antibody production) against a type-2-specific glycoprotein, G-2 (gG-2). Very few laboratories test directly for this antibody, since commercial test kits are not routinely available for this purpose. Until new tests replace the old tests, you and your physician will have to interpret information obtained very carefully. This section is an attempt to guide you through the jungle.

The *Western blot* (also called immunoblot) test has been used for diagnosis of viral infections since 1979. This test was first adapted for use with herpes simplex virus by Dr. David Bernstein in 1985. Most of the work perfecting the use of this test for clinical diagnosis has been conducted by Dr. Rhoda Ashley and her colleagues at the University of Washington. They first reported their method in 1988. Using their test, it is possible to determine from a blood sample whether a person has ever been infected with herpes simplex virus type 1, with herpes simplex virus type 2, with both, or with neither. The Western blot is by far the best understood and most reliable type-specific antibody test.

To perform a Western blot, proteins made by herpes simplex virus are separated and sorted using a technique known as electrophoresis. The viral proteins are first put on a polyacrylamide gel which resembles overly-dried Jello. By running a current through the gel, the proteins are separated into a pattern of bands unique to the viral type (herpes type 1 and type 2 have their own distinctive pattern, see figure 9).

The proteins are then transferred onto a strip of nitrocellulose

1.

The laboratory uses several different controls to be sure that a pattern is clearly specific to type 2 herpes simplex virus. Once all those criteria are met, the test is called positive. For example, if there is a predominance of binding to the type 1 strip or if there are bands of antibody bound to both strips but none are stuck to the gG-2 band (found only in type 2 virus), then there is antibody only against herpes simplex virus type 1. If there is a predominance of binding to the type 2 strip, with specific binding to the gG-2 band, then there is herpes simplex virus type 2 infection. If there is binding to both strips plus the gG-2 band, then there is probably a mixed infection (type 1 and type 2).

Highly skilled interpretation is necessary, and each specimen has to be individualized. Often several readers interpret each blot to ensure accuracy. Mixed infections (type 1 and type 2 together) are sometimes very difficult to interpret. To determine if there is any antibody to herpes simplex virus type 2 present, the laboratory may need to clear the blood sample of all of its antibody to herpes simplex virus type 1. To do this, the laboratory first mixes the sample with a purified protein mixture from type 1 virus. Any type 1 antibodies in the blood will then bind to the proteins. The mixture is then cleared from the blood and the remaining sample is retested against a herpes simplex virus type 2 strip to look for the band binding to gG-2. In this way, the laboratory expert can use a combination of patterns and other characteristics to interpret the response, minimizing the chance of a mistake.

Using these steps, there is virtually no chance of an error that shows a positive antibody to herpes simplex virus type 2 where none exists. On the other hand, there is always a small possibility that an antibody to herpes simplex virus type 2 will go undetected by this method. This could happen in the case of a recently infected person who has not yet had time to produce a lot of antibodies. In some cases, a person may take as long as twelve or sixteen weeks to develop antibodies, especially if the primary infection was treated with an effective medication. Occasionally, a person with culture-proven, long-lasting, recurrent type 2 herpes will still have a negative Western blot-presumably because they just do not make enough of the antibody. It's estimated that this occurs only about 1 percent of the time. This test is very sensitive, but does not detect every situation where genital herpes is present. In the hands of an expert laboratory, it is also very accurate, with virtually no incorrect positives made. If a person is tested more than twelve to sixteen weeks after the suspected exposure and the test is negative, then it is very likely that infection by type 2 herpes virus did not take place. However, no test is absolutely without fault. This test-like all tests-should be discussed by you and your physician in the context of all other clinical information, so that everyone understands the subtle details.

Other tests for gG-2 are also available in some research laboratories. These tests can determine whether there has been infection with herpes simplex virus type 2, but they do not determine whether there has been infection with type 1. EIA tests are technically much easier to perform than the Western blot, with much of the assay actually done by machine. Research tests of this type have been successfully used, with one described from Atlanta, one from California, another from Sweden, and an adaptation from Australia. Unfortunately, commercial ErA kit assays for antibody to gG-2 are not yet available. This situation is very likely to change soon.

For now, be especially careful to check with your physician as to which test is being ordered and how it will be interpreted. If possible, do this before being tested. The situation can be very confusing, because if your physician has ordered a so-called type-specific EIA test that does not check for antibody against gG-2 or some other type 2 viral glycoprotein, then the test may be of no value. Socalled type-specific tests that often give misleading test results are most often reported as "type 2:type 1 ratios." You may want to ask your doctor to arrange for the Western blot test instead.

It is probably best to give some examples of real cases where I have found the Western blot test to be especially useful. Test results will be different for each person depending upon their own experience. These specific examples are selected because they are particularly illustrative.

Example 1: A person with a history of genital herpes was seen twelve months after recovering from genital sores diagnosed by visual examination as probable primary genital herpes. A virus culture performed at the time was negative, but the person's physician explained that a negative result does not rule out genital herpes. At that time, the person was advised to return with an active episode for repeat culture, but no recurrences were detected. The patient has had one monogamous relationship, which started just before the so-called primary infection, with a partner who has no history of genital symptoms. They commonly practice oral-genital sex. Neither partner has cold sores.

Serology (blood antibody test) result: Both partners are positive for herpes simplex virus type 1 and negative for herpes simplex virus type 2.

Interpretation: Blood test results must be interpreted in the clinical setting. It is likely that the patient's partner does not have genital herpes. The patient's genital sores may have been a primary genital episode but, if so, probably resulted from oral-genital transmission of herpes simplex virus type 1 from the partner. Regardless, the prognosis for a continuing low genital recurrence rate is excellent. Alternatively, these blood test results could be consistent with both patient and partner having been exposed on the face to cold sores at some time in their lives, while neither has genital herpes at all. (The patient's sores may have been something else.) A third explanation is that the partner transmitted herpes simplex virus type 1 to the patient by genital contact with asymptomatic genital herpes simplex virus type 1 sores. Alternative diagnoses to the patient's primary herpes diagnosis should be considered, especially if symptoms recur frequently. The serology test is only supportive evidence for the diagnosis. It does not determine where on the body exposure has taken place, and it must be interpreted cautiously and in connection with the clinical picture. This patient with genital sores should be quite certain that other causes of genital ulcers have been ruled out, since the precise diagnosis is not yet known. In this case, the serology test has helped to rule out some things but has not specifically confirmed the clinical problem. It is very important that this patient be tested to make sure that syphilis did not cause the ulcer, since syphilitic ulcers, left untreated, will improve and then remain dormant only to cause damage later on. The result above could be consistent with both patient and partner having immunity to herpes simplex virus type 1 from asymptomatic mouth cold sores and with one partner having transmitted syphilis that has never been diagnosed or treated. Without a test, nobody will know.

Alternative serology result: Both partners are negative for both herpes simplex virus type 1 and herpes simplex virus type 2. **Interpretation:** The initial diagnosis of genital herpes was probably incorrect. An alternative diagnosis should be considered, but if the infection remains inactive, the cause may never come to light. The syphilis test discussed above is crucial, although the result is likely to be negative. If sores are recurrent, one or more specialist physicians should be involved to try to sort out the proper diagnosis.

Alternative serology result: The partner is positive for both herpes simplex virus type 1 and herpes simplex virus type 2. The patient is positive for herpes simplex virus type 2 only.

Interpretation: The initial diagnosis of genital herpes is correct. The person has had primary genital herpes simplex virus type 2 infection, and the source was probably the current partner, who is asymptomatic. Recurrences may be mild but should be expected.

Example 2: Type 2 genital herpes was proven by viral cultures in a person having a clinical first episode of genital herpes. The nontype-specific antibody test performed at the outset of this episode was positive, showing that this was a nonprimary first episode. The patient had two different sexual partners around the time of the first episode. One of the partners is interested in finding out whether he or she was the source of infection.

Serology result: The partner is positive for both herpes simplex virus type 1 and herpes simplex virus type 2.

Interpretation: The partner has genital herpes and also has been exposed to herpes simplex virus type 1. The serology test does not determine where and when the infection took place. The seropositive partner may indeed have been the source of herpes for this patient, but he or she is not the only possible source partner here. The patient could have had herpes for a while and only now be manifesting symptoms. Delving more deeply into the symptoms may help work this one out. However, most herpes is asymptomatic, so a positive test for herpes simplex virus type 2 antibody is expected more than half the time in persons with more than ten or so lifetime partners. The patient may have been positive for a long time before any contact with this current partner.

Example 3: As in example 2, type 2 genital herpes was proven in a patient with a clinical first episode. However, in this example, the early non-type-specific antibody test was negative, showing that this was a true primary first episode. Again, the patient had two different sexual partners around the time of the first episode. One of the partners is interested in finding out whether he or she was the source of infection.

Serology result: The partner is positive for herpes simplex virus type 1 and herpes simplex virus type 2.

Interpretation: This partner has exactly the same blood test results as the partner in example 2, but, in this case, the patient had a known true primary. That changes the interpretation somewhat. This partner has type 2 genital herpes and is the likely source of the primary in the patient. However, it is still possible that this partner may not have exposed the patient with primary infection. The other partner could be seropositive also and could have been the one whose herpes was active recently. In fact, it is possible that the patient with the primary could have exposed this partner to herpes for the first time, rather than the other way around. If this partner's serology test was actually taken *during* the primary infection, however, this would show that the partner was not exposed primarily to herpes by the patient, since it would take at least one or two weeks (or as long as twelve to sixteen weeks) to become seropositive.

If the story were a bit different, and the patient with the proven primary infection had had only one source partner during the month before symptoms developed, a positive serologic test for the same viral type in the partner would confirm unequivocally that the single partner was the source. However, this serology in the partner may be unnecessary, since having only one partner before developing a proven primary is strong enough evidence that that partner is the source-as long as the first clinical outbreak is actually proven to be a true primary (started out seronegative).

Now that you think you have figured this all out, think of this. It is in fact possible for a partner to be truly seronegative and transmit herpes. How? Remember that it takes a while for blood antibodies to be raised (seroconversion). If the source partner has just been infected for the first time from a different source (I.e., a different sexual partner), then he or she would not yet have converted to seropositive. In fact, people who are in the early stages of a primary infection are in their most infectious stage ever, whether or not they are showing any symptoms of herpes, since early primary infection is the time when viral shedding on mucosal surfaces is the highest.

Example 4: A patient keeps going to the physician because of recurrent genital ulcers, which look like cuts or cracks along the lines of skin folds. Cultures for herpes simplex have been taken repeatedly from sores that often have a creamy discharge. None have been positive. Simultaneous cultures of samples from the base of the sores showed only yeast on a few occasions. The physician thinks this is probably herpes but is not certain.

Serology result: The patient is negative for both herpes simplex virus type 1 and herpes simplex virus type 2.

Interpretation: This patient has no evidence of genital herpes and is probably experiencing genital ulcers because of recurrent yeast infections which require a very different type of treatment. These negative tests usually mean that there is about 99 percent chance that there has been no exposure to either herpes simplex virus type 1 or herpes simplex virus type 2. An alternative explanation is that the person was exposed less than twelve weeks ago and has not yet shown the seroconversion. There is a small (approximately 1 percent) chance that this person actually has genital herpes simplex virus type 2 herpes despite the negative serologic test. The small chance of a false negative test is likely to get even smaller in the next few years as the technology for this test continues to improve.

Example 5: A couple in a long-term relationship wish to be tested for herpes. One partner has genital herpes simplex virus type 2 proven by viral culture. The other partner is asymptomatic, although they have been together for several years. The partner wants to know if he or she is still at risk of getting genital herpes.

Serology result: There is virtually never a need to perform a Western blot in a person with viral culture proven type 2 herpes simplex virus infection, since the viral culture (if it is positive) tells you even more. That is, it identifies the infection and the site of the infection. However, the partner should be tested. In this case, she or he is seropositive for herpes simplex virus type 2.

Interpretation: This partner has genital herpes. He or she may have had genital herpes at the time the couple met, or asymptomatic transmission may have taken place at some point in their relationship. Either way, there is very little risk of the partner catching a second infection with type 2 herpes virus. This couple can relax some of their concerns about transmission of genital herpes since both already have proven infections. While there are cases of second viral strain transmission, the chance that that will occur appears to be low, although definitive studies have not been performed.

Summary

Type-specific serology testing is changing the way genital herpes is diagnosed in some cases. It is especially useful in unusual presentations of herpes and in asymptomatic cases. People with genital sores will still want to have a viral culture test from a sore for confirmation and typing. The culture test is more direct and less expensive and provides information about the sore and the symptoms. The blood test may (and often does) come up positive in people with absolutely no symptoms of genital herpes. If you have a clear positive viral culture test that is typed (type 1 versus type 2) there is almost never a reason to bother getting a Western blot also.

A negative Western blot test means that genital herpes is very unlikely, although there is still a small chance of a false negative. A positive test for type 2 herpes strongly suggests the diagnosis of genital herpes, although the test does not determine the site of infection. People with type 2 herpes infection in any site on the body will have a positive test, although most type 2 herpes is sexually transmitted and usually affects areas on or near the genitals or anus. There are obvious exceptions, however. Furthermore, since genital herpes can be caused by type 1 herpes simplex virus, a negative test for type 2 does not rule out genital herpes: it only makes type 2 genital herpes very unlikely, as long as the twelve to sixteen weeks waiting period has passed. It may take up to twelve to sixteen weeks after infection for the serology test to show positive. Any test result should be interpreted with your physician.

What type of doctor should I go to?

You may wish to start with your family doctor or internist. Find out whether your symptoms suggest herpes. If you need more detailed answers to your questions, ask to be referred to a clinic for sexually transmitted diseases or to a specialist in the area. Your physician should be able to guide you to a gynecologist, a dermatologist, a urologist, a specialist in infectious diseases, or someone Who has some special experience with herpes. It matters little how much or what type of special training the physician or health practitioner has. In some areas, it is very common for people with genital problems to go directly to a specialist; in other areas, it is common to go to a clinic, where most care is provided by a nurse or a physician's assistant. In most cases, a superspecialist is not required to get proper diagnosis, treatment, and counseling for sexually transmitted diseases. It is information and accuracy that you need. Only a trained professional can arrange for the other tests you will need to be sure you have nothing else that requires specific treatment.

Expect to be fully questioned, often about private matters. Your physician needs to know answers to (and usually needs to ask you directly) very personal questions you may never have been asked before. To provide you with some idea about the types of questions the practitioner should be asking, a questionnaire from the Viridae Herpes Clinic is included as an appendix in the back of this book. The questionnaire is for you to use if you wish when you go to your doctor. Feel free to make a copy; fill it out carefully and give it to your physician or health care provider. I am not suggesting that every health care provider should be using this same approach. The form in the appendix is for women who are pregnant. We use slightly different forms for non-pregnant women and for men. There would be additional (or different) questions we would ask in these situations, of course. However, your health care provider should be asking you at least in general terms about some of the areas covered in the questionnaire. In my opinion, the most important areas include the following:

2. Your history of herpes, including the first episode-duration, appearance, symptoms associated with it, treatment of it, tests done to determine the cause.

3. Your sexual history-Le., number of sexual partners, sexual preference, other sexually transmitted disease risk factors, risk factors for acquiring AIDS.

4. Your coping mechanisms-e.g., excessive moodiness or black moods, feeling of being depressed, thoughts about suicide, waking up during the night, thinking a lot about death.

5. Your history of other medical conditions and treatments.

6. How herpes is affecting your life in general and specifically your relationship(s).

After your physician has taken a full history about you and your herpes, you should be fully examined. A woman should have a full external and internal genital examination, at least once after the onset of her herpes (and also as a regular part of her yearly routine physical, of course). Men should be examined externally and should also, in most cases, have a urethral swab or urine test for other STDs. Examination of the area around the rectum is also important for both men and women. A full examination may not seem very dignified, but if your health care provider fails to make the right diagnosis about your infection because an examination was replaced by counseling, then you have been done no favor.

In addition to a complete history and physical examination and laboratory tests, your physician should offer specific advice about herpes. Herpes is very common, but, even today, many people with herpes find going to their doctor unsatisfactory. In a recent study from the American Social Health Association in the United States, people with herpes stated that their first health care provider had failed to take a proper sexual history or ask about personal issues in more than half of all cases!

As a health care consumer, you may need to shop around a bit, but you should get your history taken, your physical examination performed, your questions answered. Your health care provider should be comfortable with you (and you with him or her), with the diagnosis of herpes, and with your partner if you wish your partner to be present. The health care provider should arrange for follow-up if this is your primary, in order to be certain all the information and medicine did their work.

Does it matter if the herpes is type 1 or type 2?

As a general rule, herpes simplex is herpes simplex. Usually, type 1 causes oral, lip, and facial herpes, while type 2 causes genital herpes. However, type 1 may cause genital herpes and type 2 may cause oral herpes. In general, however, in North America, over 90 percent of *recurrent* genital herpes is caused by type 2. This continues to be true because type 2 herpes simplex virus infection recurs much more efficiently on the genital area compared with type 1. In part, this is probably due to the efficiency of type 2 herpes in attaching itself to nerve cells (neurons) in the sacral ganglia. In animal models, nerve cells from these areas are much easier targets for type 2 than for type 1. More sacral ganglionic neurons become latently infected and more are likely to reactivate with type 2 than with type 1.

By contrast, *primary* genital infection from a type 1 infection is very common. Primary infection results from external inoculation of skin cells from the infected skin of another. Latent infection takes place as a result. The opposite situation takes place with recurrent infection, where sores result from *reactivation* of latent neuron infection in the same person. In fact, nearly half of true primary genital herpes is now caused by type 1. Type 1 genital primaries are on the rise for a number of reasons. First of all, primary infection depends on how much virus is present in the skin of the source partner during contact. Type 1 contact potential may be increasing in adulthood because oral sex is becoming more common and is rarely a protected sexual practice (using latex barriers, for example). The vast majority of type 1 genital herpes results from unprotected oral-genital sex. Even more importantly, the level of our immunity to type 1 oral-labial herpes in adults is now much lower than it ever was. This is, of course, all the fault of our parents! They were much more aware of and careful with their cold sores than previous generations were. Their careful hygiene markedly reduced the incidence of facial type 1 herpes in children. However, these precautions have also had the side effect of leaving us significantly more susceptible to both type 1 and type 2 herpes simplex virus transmission as adults.

Therapy is now available for treatment of herpes infections.
Some of the therapy being developed may be type-specific. If typespecific therapy becomes a clinical reality (which is some time off), then typing before treatment will become absolutely necessary. Some laboratories now do herpes typing routinely. In the recent past, typing was a difficult thing to do well, but the laboratory methods for proper typing are now much easier, and they will become easier yet in the very near future.

Even before the era of type-specific therapy, however, the virus should be typed accurately during the very first episode of genital herpes. Type 1 and type 2 have very different outcomes regarding recurrence frequency and very different habits regarding methods of transmission. These differences can be quite important. For example, if a first genital outbreak occurs in a young child, the possibility of sexual abuse should be investigated by the authorities. If the child has type 1 genital herpes, it becomes possible or perhaps likely, that he or she acquired herpes through nonsexual contact. But while it is possible to conceive of a nonsexual mode of transmission for type 2 genital herpes to a child, those situations must be rare. It is also important to know your herpes type because most primary outbreaks caused by type 1 will not lead to frequent recurrences. Type 1 recurrent herpes generally occurs far less often than type 2. Thus, it is reassuring to find out during the primary episode which type you have, should it turn out to be type 1. Another reason to find out which type you have is that if it is type 1, it was probably transmitted through oral-genital contact; if so, it is likely (but not certain) that your sexual partner got herpes in a nonsexual way, because most type 1 herpes is transmitted

through mouth/facial contact in childhood. Type 1 genital herpes is also less frequently shed without symptoms compared with type 2. If transferred during childbirth to cause neonatal herpes, type 1 can cause serious infections for the neonate, but is less likely to lead to long-term problems in the infant following recovery. On the other hand, since recurrent herpes has already established its pattern, typing is often of little clinical consequence in this setting. Frequent genital herpes recurrences are almost always caused by type 2. If your current or future partner ever wishes to use the Western blot (blood) test for herpes, knowledge of the typing of your virus isolate will be very useful in interpreting the meaning of the result in your relationship.

It is also possible to tell one person's virus from another by its "DNA fingerprint" and thus to trace outbreaks of infection to their source. It seems that the possible variations from strain to strain in this virus are nearly infinite. These tools remain in the hands of researchers for now, although determination of whether your virus is type 1 or type 2 herpes is routinely available.

Genital Herpes: Transmission

How does herpes spread from person to person?

In order to infect a new host, the herpes virus must attach to the epithelial keratinocytes (skin cells). It uses its envelope to hook onto and then fuse together with the membrane of the new cell. Herpes can live only a very short time outside its host cell. Without its surrounding envelope, it dries out and is rendered sterile. Anything that dissolves the envelope, like soap or alcohol, effectively neutralizes the virus. Unlike some other viruses such as the common cold, herpes simplex virus cannot be sent across open spaces (in a room by sneezing, for example), in part because it dries out quickly. (Unlike the daring young man on the flying trapeze, herpes does not fly through the air with the greatest of ease.)

Probably a certain number of virus particles must reach epithelial cells in the new host for infection to be successful. Large numbers are necessary to compensate for the failure of most virus particles to set up effectively in their new host. Similarly, even though pregnancy results from the union of only one sperm and one egg, millions of sperm are required to ensure that one gets through to the egg. How many herpes virus particles are needed for transmission? This is unknown and will probably remain so, since the human experiment required to find the answer is not an ethical one to perform. One can easily imagine, however, that if a very small number of particles were to infect a cell, the reproduction process of the virus might lag behind the immunological defense network within the host. That network is much like an army with specialized units that have a certain starting force. Reinforcements capable of building up each battalion are always on the way. If the invasion force (the virus) is very small, no reinforcements are needed, and the invasion is quashed. If the invasion force is strong, there is a delay until reinforcements come. During the wait for reinforcements, disease occurs. Because of numbers, combined with the fact that the virus loses its ability to cause infection easily when it is outside the body for any significant period of time, direct inoculation is generally required for herpes to spread.

Direct inoculation occurs when infected epithelial cells from one person-preferably kept moist and warm at body temperature and helped by rubbing or, even better, by scratching-come in direct contact with the epithelial cells of another person. Regular skinon the hand, for example-is protected against all but the most massive invasion because of a natural barrier on the skin called *keratin.* Keratin is waxy and strong. Just as it repels water, it repels herpes virus particles (see figure 1). Unless the keratin is torn, in a cut for instance, the virus cannot get to an epithelial cell. In mucous membranes, however, like those lining the mouth, eye, and genital area, the barrier is very thin, and the epithelial cells are very near the skin surface. This is where access is easiest. On one person, there is an active lesion with herpes growing and alive; add friction for heat and for removal of infected cells from the surface of the donor; add moisture for easy travel and to prevent drying; add exposed epithelial cells of another person; and a new infection is the result.

Thus, genital herpes tends to be sexually transmitted. Other types of transmission are possible but not usual. Most friction, moisture, and heat-producing contact between two people involving the skin of the genitals is sexual. Herpes simplex can be transmitted, for example, from a penile sore to a vagina. However, transmission of genital herpes does not actually require genital penetration. Sexual contact may include a nongenital sore contacting a genital target. In other words, herpes may be transmitted from the source partner's mouth to the other partner's vagina, or from mouth to penis, penis to mouth, finger to penis, penis to anus, or any other combination. The only requirements are infected cells and exposure to new cells belonging to a new, susceptible person, along with heat and moisture. These requirements are also met in a variety of contact sports. Herpes simplex virus does not care if sex is happening. Sure, herpes likes sex, but sex is only one type of contact sport that generates heat, moisture, and frictionbased skin-to-skin contact. Herpes can be spread during wrestling, rugby, or any other contact sport that exposes a new susceptible host to infectious virus and thus provides the new environmental opportunities the virus constantly seeks to restart its reproductive cycle in a new host.

What can be done to prevent herpes from spreading?

For herpes to move from one person to another, one person must have herpes and the other person must be susceptible (not have that type of herpes). Further, these two individuals must engage in contact (usually sexual contact) during a period when virus replication is active-growing-on the skin or mucous membrane. When skin herpes is active, protection is achieved by completely avoiding sore-to-skin contact. *A condom does not offer sufficient protection against transmission when a sore is present.*

Anywhere herpes is *active* is a place to avoid having contact. If it is in the mouth, then avoid kissing, oral sex, and so on. If on the finger, keep your hand to yourself while your infection is active. If it is on your thigh, watch what rubs against your partner (try bandaging it). If it is on the genitals, during active infection avoid genital contact and consider using safer (protected) sex practices during other (asymptomatic) times. Using precautions during asymptomatic times will reduce the chance of transmission during those infrequent times when virus reactivates on the skin in very mild episodes. If an active episode is too mild to notice, it is called asymptomatic. The virus is on the skin, just not being noticed.

Herpes generally stays in specific areas of your body. For example, you need not avoid kissing if you have active genital herpes unless you have active sores on your mouth, just as people with cold sores on the mouth needn't avoid genital sex-just putting mouth-to-skin when sores are active. In other words, active herpes is a time to avoid contact with affected areas, but not a time to avoid contact altogether. In fact, it is a time for creative contact. People commonly have sexual contact during which they carefully and successfully avoid putting a finger into their sexual partner's eye. Avoiding sites of active herpes and still having sexual contact is similar. Learn to have contact while avoiding the area of skin actively affected with herpes. This is critical. Total abstinence is okay for a while, but it leads to changes in self-image that are not necessary or useful. They will be discussed later.

You think your active phases are over, but you want to offer your partner maximal protection and want to make absolutely certain that any risk of transmission caused by the small but ever-present chance of asymptomatic shedding is minimized. All people, regardless of herpes history, who have sexual contact without being committed to long-term monogamy are now strongly advised to use condoms. Many physicians also recommend the spermicidal agent *nonoxynol-9*. The latest data on the possibility of asymptomatic transmission of herpes where such protection is lacking make safer sexual practices even more compelling. All people should be taking these precautions unless they are in a monogamous, long-term relationship where the HIV status of both partners is known and there is no ongoing risk of either partner acquiring human immuno-deficiency virus from another route. In other words, if one partner in a monogamous sexual relationship continues to share needles with other drug users, his or her sexual partner remains at risk even after a negative blood test. More information on the use of condoms and safer sex techniques is given in chapter 12. During the inactive phases of infection, protected sex using latex condoms will reduce the small risk of transmission and enhance your peace of mind. If your symptoms are over, chances are you've got no virus left on the skin. If you have, chances are it is a small amount. Should asymptomatic shedding occur while you are using condoms properly (see chapter 12), the chances of avoiding transmission are strongly in your favor. A study published in the *Journal of*

Infectious Diseases followed couples over sixteen months where one partner had genital herpes and the other did not (determined by the Western blot test). Asymptomatic transmission did take place in some patients in this study; however, none of the couples in whom asymptomatic transmission took place regularly used safer sex practices.

Some people find that in the beginning-for the first several months after their initial herpes-telling one phase from the next is tricky. Regardless of how you perceive your symptoms, however, in the six months or so following a true primary infection, asymptomatic shedding of herpes is especially common. With careful attention to your body during this period, an awareness generally comes easily. You will get to know your herpes with time. During your getting-to-know period, properly used latex condoms ensure a very low risk of transmission to your partner. If herpes is a new thing in your relationship, however, you will also want to determine with certainty whether your partner has herpes also. If your partner does not have herpes already, then he or she remains at risk of getting it, thus increasing the need for safer sex during the post-primary period. If you have had a true primary infection with type 2 herpes while you were monogamous, however, and you continue to be with the same monogamous partner, there is a reasonable chance that both of you already have genital herpes, regardless of your partner's symptoms or lack thereof. In this case, you would be best advised to determine with your health care provider(s) whether both of you already have herpes. In the meantime, while you are waiting for a reliable answer to this important question, you can always take the position of assuming that your partner is still susceptible to infection. With apologies to Benjamin Franklin, better safe than sorry.

To avoid both herpes and AIDS, careful use of quality latex condoms as a safer sex practice is always recommended. Once both you and your partner understand the risks of getting sexually transmitted diseases (STDs) including AIDS and genital herpes, you can determine how to proceed based on accurate information.

I have herpes on my buttocks (or thigh or foot). How did it get there? Did I spread it from my genitals to this other spot?

This question is an extremely common and important one. If one area on your body can be affected, why not everywhere? Can herpes move around? Herpes sticks to infection of the skin and the local sensory nerves that supply the specific area affected. It does not get tossed around from organ to organ. Herpes is extremely stable in the general area supplied with those nerves. In fact, stability is one of the characteristics that makes herpes so difficult to cure. It gets in one place and sticks with it. There may be a slight variation of the precise skin site from one recurrence to another. This results from the branching of nerve fibers. Herpes strictly follows the nerve to the skin-even if it branches off in a new direction. On one occasion, for example, a herpes reactivation may originate inside one neuron in the ganglion whose nerve fiber supplies a small spot of genital skin of the right side. These nerve fibers have precise routes to the skin and the virus is just as bound to stick with the appointed route as a train is bound to stick to its tracks. It simply cannot veer from its route back to the original skin site any more than electricity can leave the wire on its way from the socket to the lamp, unless a predetermined branch in the tracks or the wire is present.

Therefore, when herpes recurs in a new spot also supplied by the same neural network from the sacral ganglia, you can be certain that the virus did not spill from its tracks. Rather, the reactivating ganglionic cell has a route to the skin that branches elsewhere. This cell could be right next to the cell whose branches go directly to the genitals. In the central switching house of the sacral plexus, cells close enough to be simultaneously infected with latent herpes may lead to related but widely separated areas of skin at the other end of the nerve's branches. Thus, a subsequent "genital" herpes recurrence may find itself in a slightly different area-for example, the buttocks.

Buttock herpes is an interesting and very understudied entity, in general. Probably about 10 percent of people with symptomatic genital herpes get buttock sores sometimes also. Only about 50 percent of people with episodes of buttock herpes are aware of their genital symptoms, but herpes is *almost never* directly inoculated or indirectly autoinoculated to the buttocks. Herpes on the buttocks is a classic demonstration of the nerve branching phenomenon just described. Reactivations emanating from neighboring sacral ganglionic neurons are apparently "wired" to both genital and buttock skin.

So, is buttock herpes the same as genital herpes? Of course, buttocks are not genitals. No, there has not been a recent surge of buttock sex in our society. Nor has there been a new wave of people catching buttock herpes from toilet seats. Buttock herpes is one possible clinical manifestation of genital herpes, because of this nerve tracking business. Many people only get their "genital" herpes on the buttock or thigh or even on the bottom of the foot. As far as we know, people with herpes on the buttock at some point also had genital herpes. That is how the virus got to the neuron that reactivated and branched to the buttock/thigh/foot skin. This may be even more surprising for some people whose lesions feel and look very different when they appear in different spots. So, most sexually transmitted herpes in non genital skin is not autoinoculated (spread from one part of a person's body to another part) at all. Rather, herpes is following its nerve tracks to alternative routes.

What about true autoinoculation? Can I accidentally spread genital herpes into my eyes? My brain?

People are often concerned about whether they are going to accidentally move this virus all over themselves or to a vital organ by mistake. If, during an active period, you broke a herpes vesicle (blister) with a needle and stuck the needle into your arm, your eye, your lip, or even your brain, for that matter, you probably would develop a new infection at that new site. Injection of herpes from one individual's cold sore into the same individual's arm was actually tested (questionable by today's ethical standards) on prisoner "volunteers" several decades ago. I have had one patient in my clinic who accidentally performed this experiment on himself. He thought that breaking herpes blisters with a needle might help them to heal. (He was mistaken.) Unfortunately, he once slipped and stuck his finger with the needle after breaking his blisters. Now he has herpes recurring on his finger. Aside from such extreme circumstances, however, herpes very rarely winds up moving from one site to another.

Another person I've seen gets recurrent cold sores, usually on the corner of his nose. One August, during an active outbreak, the pollen was heavy in the air. His hay fever was in full bloom along with the flowers. He sneezed and sneezed. He rubbed his itchy eyes and rubbed some more. Later, herpes sores appeared on his eyelids. While this is an example of type 1 autoinoculation, the general principles are the same as for type 2. Extreme circumstances can occasionally result in autoinoculation.

In general, however, autoinoculation is very uncommon after the primary infection is over and the person's immune system has been established against herpes simplex. The immune system prevents most accidental attempts at autoinoculation that might occur from absentmindedness. That does not mean that reasonable personal hygiene is not a good idea. It is only that nature has taken many opportunities to protect us from our own carelessness, making autoinoculation unlikely. During the primary infection, before the immune system is fully established against this virus, autoinoculation is possible. However, the fact that genital herpes is generally held within the confines of underwear means that there is even more protection against this problem.

Autoinoculation to a distant body site (for example, the fingers) is much more likely to occur during the initial attack, especially if it is a true primary. This may occur in up to 10 percent of true primary cases. During this period, immune defenses such as antibodies and lymphocytes are not yet operating at full steam, and therefore little obstruction lies in the path of virus that is anxious to move on to new places using the classical travel characteristics of friction, heat, moisture, and sore-to-skin contact. Immunity will largely prevent the virus from spreading, so, once the primary episode is over, the amount of virus required for new sores to take root is much higher. Immunity alone, however, is not enough of a defense against a lot of virus.

Good hygiene is a good idea. But don't get carried away. Instead of good hygiene, perhaps the word should be reasonable hygiene. Think about what you are doing when you touch your sores. Wash your hands afterwards. Keep contact lenses out of your mouth the same way you should keep them away from your genitals. If sores are active, don't wipe your genitals and then rub your face with the same cloth. Even if you do such a thing, you probably won't have a problem, but why do it? Transmission to your eyes from your own genitals is talked about often but almost never seen. Of several thousand patients I have seen with genital herpes, only two have had type 2 eye infections. Herpes may have been inoculated there at the same time it was inoculated onto the genitals. Autoinoculation in that situation is unlikely. Genital herpes is not a blinding disease. Herpes of the eye is usually caused by type 1. Generally, that infection is transmitted from the mouth of one person to the face of the susceptible other. Often this occurs from parent to child. The ganglion of facial herpes is called the trigeminal ganglion. The trigeminal nerve supplies sensation to the face through three divisions: mandibular, maxillary, and ophthalmic. The mandibular branch supplies the lower third of the face, the maxillary branch the middle third, and the ophthalmic branch the upper third. Usually, herpes sets up its latent infection in the lower two-thirds-the mandibular or maxillary eye divisions. Cold sores around the mouth are accounted for by those divisions. If, however, the ophthalmic branch of the nerve is infected-e.g., through a kiss to the upper third of the face-then herpes simplex virus will establish latent infection in the ophthalmic division of the trigeminal ganglion. Recurrences from there will follow their appointed "train tracks" and often end up inside the eye. A person can accomplish this with type 2 herpes from the genitals of a partner; it is just a bit more difficult, often involving a slight degree of contortion ism. This is not a common clinical problem. Fortunately, ophthalmic (eye) herpes infections in general are getting much easier to treat and suppress with the advent of good antiviral medications.

Genital herpes autoinoculated to the brain is another matter.
Rare cases of such events in severely immunologically compromised patients have been reported. Such events are rare even in patients who are severely immunologically compromised. It is safe to say, in general, that encephalitis, or brain infection, is no more likely to happen to the person with genital herpes than it is to anyone else. It is rare, still a bit confusing to scientists as to how and why it happens in the first place, difficult to treat, and extremely dangerous. There is no association at all with genital herpes in

adults. Yes, herpes simplex virus type 2 can affect the nervous system. Type 2 herpes can even cause herpes encephalitis, but it does so only extremely rarely in adults. Type 2 herpes of the newborn, however, does cause encephalitis in a small proportion of affected babies (see chapter 6). Frequently, though, type 2 genital herpes causes an inflammation of the protective sac around the brain called the meninges. The inflammation is called *aseptic meningitis* and commonly accompanies a true primary of genital herpes. Meningitis does not damage the brain or you. It can cause a severe headache and/or a stiff neck, however (see chapter 3), and it makes some people temporarily very moody and sensitive to bright lights. Nongenital herpes infections are discussed in chapter 10.

Can I transmit oral herpes to my own genitals?

Could you give yourself genital herpes by rubbing a sore on your mouth and then touching your own genitals? During primary infection in children, this may actually be common. A child with primary oral herpes (usually called gingivostomatitis) who is frequently moving hands from mouth to teething ring to genitalia and back may develop genital sores. These sores are generally type 1 and are seen in the context of a primary facial infection in the child too young to understand disease prevention. Remember, though, this child with primary infection is *non immune.* An adult is very unlikely to have this type of problem in this way. The average adult is less likely to get primary mouth infection and is also less frequently going to move his/her hands directly from mouth to genitalia.

Most often when these questions are asked, however, the person has fully recovered from the primary infection and has virtually no problem with autoinoculation. In this case, the immune system is the first protection and is very unlikely to let a second infection through. People who get cold sores often wonder whether they might transmit oral herpes to the genitals of their sexual partner and then become reinfected with their own virus (now their partner's also) back onto their own genitals through genital sex. It is theoretically possible, although extremely rare, for this sequence of events to occur. First, the viral dose required is probably very high. In this case, the person is protected by his or her own immunity against his or her own specific virus. It must be possible, however, for the same reason that the prisoner volunteers described earlier developed sores in the arm. They were immune already, but when enough virus was inoculated by needle into the arm, sores developed. In this case, the transmission method would be sexual, instead. I believe I have seen this occur once or twice in practice, although it must be very rare and difficult to document.

During primary genital herpes, however, autoinoculation is much more readily produced. Local inoculation from one place to another right next to it is normal during the primary. For example, vaginal secretions naturally spread over the perineum, where new sores may develop before your body has developed strong immunity to herpes, which takes a couple of weeks after the first infection starts. Herpes cannot jump from place to place on its own, but if enough virus is put directly into a new place, a new infection may occur.

Can I spread herpes without sexual intercourse-e.g., to my children?

Direct contact is required in order to contract herpes-not necessarily sexual contact. If your child's skin touches your herpes, then of course it can spread. In fact, most herpes simplex virus infections begin during childhood when the baby or child is kissed by a relative or friend with active type 1 herpes on her or his mouth. In general, babies are kissed on the face, but babies may also be (lovingly and appropriately) kissed in all sorts of strange places. I am sure you have seen a doting parent burying their face into the belly button area of a young baby from time to time. Often such strange human activities take place with the expression of unusual and often unrepeatable silly noises from the adult with responsive gurgling, babbling, and laughing from the recipient infant. These "contact sports" keep cropping up all over the place if you really go looking for them.

Objects that pass quickly from one person to another are, theoretically, a possible source of transmission as well. For example, if you share a drinking cup or a cigarette while you have a cold sore, transmission is possible. This is almost certainly a significant source of transmission in families. How about lipstick sharing? You bet. I often wonder how cosmetic counters can allow multiple lipstick testers. Probably, this is not a bigger problem because of the time between customers and whatever little magic the salesperson performs with a cloth. How about bath towels and genital herpes, though? Yes, I would suggest not sharing towels with others while lesions are active. That would logically go for underwear and other intimate articles. I am willing to wager, however, that fewer people share underwear than lipstick. For a lot of reasons not related to herpes, we do not tend to share things quickly from one person to another that involve intimate touching of genital skin in both persons. Furthermore, washing towels and other articles with plain soap dissolves the herpes envelope and kills the virus effectively. There is no need to use special disinfectants or virus killers. I have not seen any good evidence that sharing of bath articles has ever caused one case of herpes. But why risk it? Not sharing bath articles seems a small price to pay! Despite lots of headlines about towels, toilet seats, articles in doctors' offices, and even hot tubs and water slides, no evidence for transmission in these ways has been found. The best evidence is that children are not flocking to physicians with genital herpes. Patients with genital herpes generally avoid giving genital herpes to their children because they do not have sexual contact with their children. It is that simple. That is not to imply that rare exceptions do not exist, because they probably do. You need do no more for prevention, however, than to use reasonable personal hygiene.

What about toilet seats?

The toilet seat argument has been around since toilet seats were invented. Researchers have looked for many diseases, including gonorrhea and syphilis, on toilet seats. Herpes that gets onto a toilet seat, especially a wet, warm one that has not been cleaned in a few days, can stay alive there for quite some time. It does not stay very healthy. It begins to die as soon as it leaves the skin, but it takes a while. If the toilet seat is dried or cleaned, the herpes disappears. If the seat stays wet, the herpes may take an hour or two to fizzle. However, if herpes were alive on the seat, transmission to the next person by this method would still be unlikely, because toileting is not enough of a contact sport. The back of the thigh and the buttocks are thick-skinned areas, relatively resistant to penetration by virus. They are common sites for recurrences, because of the branching of the sensory nerves of the area down to these sites, but the temperature and moisture settings on toilet seats are all wrong for direct transmission to those sites, although nothing is impossible. I have not seen or heard of proven cases of genital herpes from toilet seats or from any other inanimate objects (swimming pools, saunas, water slides). Aside from the lack of friction, moisture, and heat, there are several other reasons which make these sources unlikely. In the case of toilet seats, most public facilities are disinfected regularly with industrial-strength disinfectants that linger on dirty seats and kill germs, herpes included. An experiment suggested that herpes could survive for a few hours on a non-disinfected toilet seat. The authors concluded that maybe toilet seats could serve as a possible source for herpes. However, experiments have never provided any evidence whatsoever for actual transmission by this route. I interpret these findings to show that toilet seats that are not disinfected do not actively kill the virus. Instead, the virus dies slowly on its own. My conclusion from the same data? Do not try to kill your herpes by banging it with a toilet seat, disinfected or otherwise.

I have spent a lot of time on toilet seats in my life and have often wondered how a sexually transmissible virus could get onto the seat in the first place. Certainly if sores are present at the bottom of the buttocks or on the back of the thigh, then those sores will touch the seat. I do recommend that people with sores in those places use toilet paper or seat covers while the sores are in their active phases. They might consider drying off the seat for others, or using a pocket-sized wet napkin. If your sores are on the penis, the labia, the pubic area, or the mouth, the problem is avoided by keeping those areas away from contact with the seat. This seems straightforward to me. The overwhelming majority of people with genital sores never contact the seat with their sores unless they have unusual personal habits. A now late colleague of mine, upon reading in the newspaper about the toilet seat issue, suggested that herpes is transmitted in public toilets only when two people make love in the stall!

No, there should not be separate toilets for people with herpes.

My personal bias and infectious disease background suggest that daily disinfection of toilets is a good idea and that toilet seat covers are not a bad commodity. However, these suggestions will help to prevent infectious hepatitis, viral diarrheas, and typhoid fever much more than syphilis or herpes. I remain shocked, as an infectious disease specialist, at how frequently men do not wash their hands after using public facilities. This is the one place in this book where I have limited myself to discussing one gender, since I can honestly say that I do not frequent facilities for women and therefore have no data. We continue to see restaurant-based outbreaks of hepatitis and other bad things that sometimes get into the food from the hands of sloppy cooks. For herpes, though, the toilet seat issue is almost an academic one.

Can I have herpes without having sores?-Asymptomatic shedding

First, the word asymptomatic must be defined. Asymptomatic can mean different things, depending upon the situation. For example, we already know that most people who have genital herpes do not know that fact. These people are all asymptomatic, in the sense that they do not recognize their symptoms and have never realized that they have genital herpes. We also know that if an accurate blood test is used to diagnose herpes in these people (for example, positive type 2 Western blot), and if they are then provided with proper education and counseling and informed of the often subtle and atypical presentations of herpes lesions, then the majority of so-called asymptomatic people with herpes will easily learn within a few months to recognize their symptoms and their active phases of infection.

For people who know about their herpes, however, the issues are different. The question is whether a person can have active herpes virus replication somewhere in or on the genital tract while experiencing nothing at all that suggests an active phase of infection.

This person has had herpes enough times to recognize and understand its active phases and the end of the active phases that comes with the onset of full skin healing. After this point, the chances of recovering virus from the skin through any kind of test are markedly reduced during asymptomatic periods. Asymptomatic shedding (the appearance of virus on the skin without symptoms) occurs on approximately 1 to 5 percent of days, precise results depending on a number of factors that vary from study to study. Several clinical studies have now shown that asymptomatic people with genital herpes who are frequently tested or swabbed for herpes by viral culture during fully healed or asymptomatic phases will have virus on the skin occasionally, when it is not expected. It is entirely normal for this to happen to people with herpes, even people who clearly understand their active phases of infection and people who are being very careful about avoiding sore-to-skin contact during active phases. Presumably, when unexpected virus is found in a study, a very mild episode must be occurring right at that moment that would otherwise go unnoticed.

In many episodes that are thought to be asymptomatic, there are actually symptoms that have not been recognized as herpes. A hemorrhoid that suddenly swells up and itches is usually just a hemorrhoid; occasionally, however, it could be a reactivation of perianal herpes. In fact, studies suggest that asymptomatic herpes is most common in the area around the anus, a very difficult area to see. Intermittent pain in the leg could be a herpes prodrome. An itch in the pubic hair is probably a pimple or just an itch; if there is a little sore behind some hair, however, it could be herpes. The list is endless. This all really means the same old thing: get to know your herpes. Be aware of where your herpes is likely to occur, and avoid contact when an unusual symptom arises there. Wait and see. Do blisters or ulcers (even very small ones) ever develop? If not, your itch is probably just an itch.

The risk of having herpes on the skin when you do not have any symptoms is not great on any specific day, but there is still a definite risk. Dr. Vontver and his coworkers in Seattle studied pregnant women's risk of having a no-symptoms, no-sores, culture-positive recurrence. In the absence of visible lesions, herpes was isolated in 7 of 1,068 cervical cultures (0.66 percent) and 8 of 1,068 external genital cultures (0.75 percent). Another study of pregnant women, by Dr. 1. H. Harger and coworkers in Pittsburgh, suggested an asymptomatic rate of virus shedding of about 3 percent. A Vancouver study showed asymptomatic shedding numbers in late pregnancy at about 4 percent. Numbers depend on a number of factors. For example, the immune system may be different in late pregnancy than at other times. Pressure on the vulva from the fetus may alter the rate of recurrences or even make detection more difficult. Yeast infections common in late pregnancy may be easily confused with herpes. In addition, studies vary depending upon how well the subjects undergoing study know the characteristics of their herpes. The sensitivity of the laboratory (how much virus is necessary to get a positive test) may be important, as well as the care of the physician responsible for looking for sores (is this really asymptomatic or missed symptomatic?). In another study, by Dr. S. Straus and his associates from the National Institutes of Health, twenty-six volunteers with frequent genital herpes (but not pregnant or ill in any way) underwent daily genital cultures. Asymptomatic shedding over eleven months occurred in 8 per 1,000 cultures. This accounted for 28 asymptomatic episodes in 26 people, each asymptomatic episode lasting an average of 1.54 days. So asymptomatic genital herpes shedding happens-just not very often and not for very long.

Asymptomatic shedding is more common soon after the primary infection. In fact, for three months after a true primary type 2 infection, cervical asymptomatic shedding is present on about 17 percent of routine visits! Asymptomatic shedding after primary type 1 genital herpes is much lower than after primary type 2. Despite the infrequency and short time span of asymptomatic shedding, recent data suggest that nearly everyone with type 2 herpes has very short, asymptomatic shedding periods every so often.

A recent study by Dr. Anna Wald and her colleagues from the University of Washington followed 110 women very closely for symptoms and viral shedding. This study uses the term "subclinical shedding," defined as all of the active phases of an infection in which a sore is present. Thus, a person who shed virus in this study during a prodromal or warning phase was still identified as subclinical. Over a three-and-a-half-month period, approximately half of the women with type 2 herpes shed virus subclinically. About 29 percent of those with type 1 did so. Women with type 2 herpes shed virus subclinically on approximately 2 percent of the days. The average duration of the shedding period was a day and a half. A common site for subclinical shedding of virus was around the anus. The genital skin, perineum, and cervix were also sites of shedding. In general, the more symptomatic recurrences a woman experienced in this study, the more subclinical recurrences she also experienced. Recent studies show, however, that even people with no history of symptoms of genital herpes will experience subclinical shedding (if they have genital herpes). In fact, it would appear that of the total number of days where virus can be grown from a swab of these areas, about one-third to one-half of those shedding days are identified by the person with herpes as subclinical. This study again showed that the frequency of shedding without signs seemed to decrease somewhat with time. However, this same research group has more recently shown that a person who tends to shed subclinically frequently at one point in time tends to do the same a few years later.

As technology improves, so does our ability to detect herpes when shedding occurs. Over the past few years, Drs. Anna Wald and Larry Corey have aggressively and carefully studied the topic of asymptomatic viral shedding using standard viral cultures, along with a new technique called the *polymerase chain reaction* (PCR). Herpes PCR is so sensitive that it can detect a few molecules of viral hereditary material (DNA) in a swab. (pCR is famous for identification of blood stains during criminal investigationsremember the O. J. Simpson trial?) Using PCR techniques, Drs. Wald and Corey and others have found that herpes DNA can be present in small quantities on the skin far more often than was ever found with viral culture alone. These studies suggest that herpes may reactivate more frequently than has ever been realized before. Apparently, our immune systems are very capable of quickly shutting off herpes when it reactivates. Herpes reactivates from its latent site regularly, but most often the immune response shuts these reactivations off before any living virus makes its way to the skin surface. When the peR test comes up positive, most of the time there is no surviving virus left-just its peR fingerprint. The immune system has seen to that. Occasionally, the peR test and the culture test come up positive at the same time.

peR may be used as a diagnostic test, because it will not be positive in someone who does not have herpes. When peR is used to examine for asymptomatic herpes, however, it comes up positive more than 20 percent of the time. What does that mean? The answers are not in yet. While a PfR test cannot be positive in a person without herpes, it can be positive in a person who does have herpes at times where no symptoms are present and no living virus is present on the skin. For now, peR is an intriguing research tool that will greatly aid in understanding the reactivation process of genital herpes. Since a positive PfR test is common without any living virus, however, it is not entirely clear what it means on a clinical basis. In certain clinical situations, the peR test has already shown itself to be quite useful for the very reason that it will detect even a remaining fingerprint of the virus. Research in this area will definitely be something to watch carefully.

What are the chances that asymptomatic viral shedding might lead to asymptomatic transmission to my sexual partner?

Two key clinical studies have examined transmission risks in couples. Much more data will become known in the next few years as results from herpes vaccine studies become available. We do know a few key facts. Most people who transmit herpes to their partner do so while they are in an asymptomatic phase of infection. This makes sense, since people do whatever they can to avoid having sexual contact with the affected area while they are in an active phase of infection. Dr. Gregory Mertz and his colleagues followed 144 heterosexual couples for 334 days for evidence of transmission from one person to the other. These investigators were studying a vaccine which turned out to be completely ineffective. The couples were counseled about the active phases of infection and advised to avoid skin-to-skin contact during those phases. They were further advised to use safer sex practices during asymptomatic periods, but only IS percent of the couples did so regularly. Herpes infections were assessed by the usual methods of diagnosis, including symptoms, cultures, and Western blots. Of 144 sexual partners who were susceptible to herpes, 14 (9.7 percent) acquired infection during this study. In 9 of the 14 cases, no recent symptoms or signs of herpes were reported by the person who transmitted herpes. In 4 of the 14 cases, active phases of infection were reported either during or just after sexual intercourse. In one case, no information was available.

This study showed that the greatest risk for acquiring genital herpes from a partner was based on gender. Women were more than four times as likely as men to acquire genital herpes. In addition to gender, another risk factor was the absence of previous type 1 herpes. More than half of the people in this study (like more than half of the population in general) had antibody to type 1 herpes. People who had no antibody to type 1 herpes acquired genital herpes a little over twice as often as people who had previous type 1 antibody (with or without a history of cold sores). Women who had no antibody to type 1 herpes acquired genital herpes three-and-a-half times more often than women who had type 1 antibody. In this study, couples who regularly used safer sex practices acquired herpes 58 percent less than those who did not. Unfortunately, because so few practiced safer sex regularly, these differences were not found to be statistically significant.

In a separate study from Los Angeles, Dr. Yvonne Bryson studied 57 heterosexual couples where one partner had type 2 genital herpes and the other partner felt that he or she did not. She found that 19 percent of the partners who thought they did not have genital herpes at the start of the study actually did, so they were not counted in the results. The couples were also educated about herpes and about transmission and then followed for approximately 16 months. In this study, the annual rate of transmission (I.e. the proportion of individuals who acquired the herpes virus in one year) to women was 22 percent. For women with no antibody to type 1 herpes, the annual rate was about 32 percent, while it was 16 percent in women who had pre-existing antibody to type 1. Half of the women in this study who acquired type 2 herpes had known, unprotected exposures to active phases of infection in their partners. In this study, none of the men acquired herpes at all. Most of the transmissions occurred early in the relationship, while many couples who had been together for years continued to avoid transmission. Finally, transmission did not occur in any of the couples who regularly used safer sex practices.

These studies demonstrate many important things. First of all, it is impossible in long-term relationships to *completely* eliminate the risk of transmitting genital herpes. While it is not fully proven, there is little doubt that safer sex practices will help to reduce the risks quite substantially. Remember, safer sex practices with herpes means having no skin-to-skin contact with the affected area during the active phases of infection and using condoms properly (see chapter 12) during asymptomatic times. These studies also show that there is reason to hope that a herpes vaccine will someday help to reduce transmission rates, since, in some studies, type 1 herpes antibody itself seems to protect people from getting herpes by at least a factor of two. Furthermore, women are at much higher risk of getting herpes from their male partners than vice versa. Some of the transmissions were avoidable by being careful with active phases, but some were not. It is for those times that safer sex practices can playa very helpful role.

When making choices about preventing herpes transmission, it is clearly wise to consider the possibility that asymptomatic shedding may occur. In case asymptomatic shedding does occur, safer sex practices including proper use of condoms are the best way to minimize the low everyday risk that asymptomatic shedding may lead to asymptomatic transmission. Using sensitive and strict criteria for identifying people acquiring herpes, the University of Washington study showed that simply avoiding sexual contact during the active phases of infection provides enough protection for more than 95 percent of susceptible men and more than 81 percent of susceptible women per year. Both studies clearly showed, however, that simple avoidance during active phases alone is not sufficient to completely prevent transmission. To further minimize the risk of transmission to a susceptible partner, safer sex practices should be used during asymptomatic periods. Be careful, also, about interpreting the word susceptible here. For these studies, susceptible meant that the partner of a person with type 2 genital herpes had no Western blot antibody to type 2 herpes at the beginning of the study period. This is not at all the same as the situation where one person in the relationship has no history of herpes. Western blot antibody to type 2 herpes is present in at least one of five people who have no history of genital herpes. If a person already has Western blot antibody to type 2 herpes, he or she is at minimal risk, from that point on, of acquiring any new type 2 herpes infection from a person with type 2 herpes. He or she may have originally been infected by you or by a different person, depending on the circumstances, but second infections with second strains of type 2 herpes are very uncommon. Second infections are possible, but if a partner who has Western blot antibody to type 2 herpes develops clinical herpes, chances are that any clinical infection in that person will result from their own herpes reactivating.

With all this information about asymptomatic shedding and asymptomatic transmission, what should I do about it?

What have these studies shown us? On the one hand, when looking at the number of days of the year affected, the risk of asymptomatic shedding is really quite low. There is, however, a continuously present, small statistical chance of coming in contact with an active, unsuspected episode of genital herpes. In many long-term partnerships, transmission will not take place even over a period of years. With the passage of time, however, the herpes roulette wheel keeps spinning and small chances build up to significant ones. With each spin of the wheel, the chances remain very low in careful people. Safer sex improves the odds significantly in favor of protection. Don't forget that genital herpes is so common, and so often completely unknown to people who have it, that the everyday roulette wheel of life in the 90s makes the chance of getting herpes from any sexual partner extremely high. It is very common that people who think they do not have herpes actually have it. Type 2 herpes is present in approximately 20 percent of Vancouver women who have had at least one sexual partner and in 55 percent of women who have had at least 10 sexual partners. In the United States, genital herpes may be even more common, with asymptomatic seropositivity rates of up to 30 percent overall in private practice gynecology clinics. Herpes transmission is probably just as likely to occur if one partner thinks he or she does not have herpes and really does have it as it is if he or she knows and is being careful-especially if being careful includes safer sex practices.

In the future, both vaccines and drugs may play an important role in preventing herpes transmission (see chapter 11). Recent studies have also proven that antiviral medications (acyclovir, tamciclovir, valacyclovir) taken at least twice daily on a continuous basis (dosing of medicine is something to decide with your doctor) will reduce asymptomatic viral shedding by as much as 75 to 90 percent depending upon the circumstances. Studies are under way to determine if blocking asymptomatic shedding will also block transmission to partners. In general, transmission studies are more difficult to perform. They are very expensive and require the longterm participation of couples in relationships. It is not a big scientific leap, though, to think that if a treatment reduces asymptomatic shedding by 80 percent or more, it might very well reduce transmissions from this shedding as well. If you decide to use treatments to reduce asymptomatic shedding, please note that this is not yet officially approved by regulatory authorities. You should discuss the issues with your doctor carefully before proceeding.

For some partners, the information about risks of transmission is not enough to reassure them. Sometimes, people with herpes worry too much about the potential for transmission. The situation is made worse if the person is very uncomfortable about talking about herpes with partners. A high level of concern and care regarding sexual practices-including limiting the number of partners, using safer sex precautions, and discussing herpes-is now necessary. That is today's reality. *Avoidance of sexual contact altogether because of herpes* is *not called for under any circumstance.* If you find yourself doing that, however, you are not alone. Many people avoid relationships altogether, in order to keep their herpes secret. Others limit contacts to casual partners in order to avoid discussing it. In either case, the secret itself has become the problem. It is best to begin to undo herpes-caused celibacy as soon as possible. Find a doctor who is comfortable with your problem and who offers specific suggestions for you. If necessary, go for counseling to get your feelings about this sorted out. Share your feelings confidentially with a close friend. Herpes continues to increase in frequency mostly because people are unaware of their infection. You can be very effective at minimizing transmission risk through straightforward rules. It is wise to choose your sexual partner carefully, but staying alone with your secret will not help you or the rest of the world. Approximately 75 percent of all people who have genital herpes do not think they have it and thus, thinking there is no problem, continue to have unprotected sexual contact, with mild sores going unnoticed. Despite all the studies of asymptomatic shedding, the usual source partners of first episodes of genital herpes are people who do not think they have herpes. In other words, the vast majority of partners of people with first episodes of genital herpes are people who thought they did not have genital herpes.

Thus, avoiding sexual contact with a careful person who has herpes may not be an effective means of avoiding this virus. Asking people if they have herpes is also an ineffective test, since most people who have herpes think they don't. A sexual partner who denies having genital herpes could place you at a higher risk of infection than a partner who knows how to avoid transmission of a known and identifiable entity. If your partner has genital herpes and you are susceptible, you are not free of risk, though. You may wish to determine your susceptibility through the Western blot test. If that test shows you to be susceptible, you and your partner are advised to use safer sex practices to decrease the chance of asymptomatic transmission. Stay informed about the availability of vaccines or vaccine studies in your area. Early results from one of the candidate vaccines have been disappointing but additional studies are ongoing. If either you or your partner has a high risk factor for HIV, you may want to get counseling about HIV and be tested for it also, so you and your partner will be in a better position to decide about giving up safer sex practices. If you do not have herpes, though, and you are looking for guarantees that you won't get herpes now or in the future, forget it. The only way to be sure of this is to avoid all sexual contact with all people, regardless of their herpes history, forever.

In summary, regarding the issues of transmission of herpes to a partner, consider the following:

1. Discuss your herpes openly and frankly with your partner before having sexual contact.

2. If your partner has no recollection of having herpes, but has had previous sexual partners, consider asking your health care provider for a Western blot test for your partner to find out whether he or she already has asymptomatic herpes of the same type.

3. Get to know your herpes and avoid all skin-to-skin contact with affected areas during active phases of infection. During active phases you may wish to use sexual techniques that do not include contact with your active areas.

4. Learn about safer sex practices and use them every time you have sexual contact with your partner. After you have all the information and both you and your partner understand the issues, you can decide together about how you want to handle the safer sex issues for the longer term.

5. Discuss with your doctor the possibility of using antiviral suppression to reduce the frequency of asymptomatic shedding, if that appeals to you and your partner. This is not an absolute prevention method, but it does reduce the frequency of shedding substantially. Used in conjunction with the other methods discussed here, it may playa role for you.

6. Find out about the status of vaccinations for herpes. Your doctor or clinic may be participating in clinical trials or know more about one of the new vaccines under study.

If I have herpes, am I immune to a second infection from someone else?

Not fully and completely, but for most practical purposes. A study done in 1980 in Atlanta, Georgia, showed that genital herpes can

recur with more than one strain of the virus. People with one strain of herpes can get another. Since immunity is important, it is generally thought that getting herpes a second time is substantially more difficult than getting it the first time. In the section on autoinoculation, a similar question is raised-Le., can I give herpes to myself in a new place? Transmission of type 2 genital herpes to a person who has Western blot antibody against type 2 herpes is rare. Studies have shown that a person with genital herpes can catch a new case of genital herpes, but other studies have shown that this happens only rarely. In most cases, if a person with genital herpes catches genital herpes while with a partner, they are catching it from themselves (having a recurrence). Type-specific antibody against your own strain of virus makes it very difficult to catch a second infection from a different person.

It takes painstaking effort to tell one herpes strain from another, but it can be done. The test is not one a family doctor or even a specialist can perform. In order to tell the herpes of Mr. Jones from the herpes of Ms. Smith, a "DNA fingerprint" is obtained: the virus is grown in the laboratory and purified, and the DNA (see chapter 1) is extracted with chemicals. Then, enzymes called restriction endonucleases are added, which cut the DNA in several special places. The small pieces that are left are put into a wobbly but firm gel and an electric charge is introduced, causing the pieces to travel inside the gel. This test bears some similarity to the Western blot test, in which small proteins travel inside a gel. In this case, the travelers are small pieces of DNA. Since small pieces travel faster than large ones, the gel makes a "fingerprint." Using this method, researchers have shown subtle differences between the fingerprints of different virus strains. Rarely, two strains on separate recurrences in the same person and dual infections of two strains at the same time have been observed. However, second infections with new strains are considered to be extremely rare. Studies that have sought different strains from a single person with genital herpes have had a very difficult time finding them in most people. Yet statistics suggest that people with genital herpes commonly come in contact with herpes more than from more than one partner. There must be a very strong immunity to second infection, although it is not yet defined scientifically. Although incomplete, immunity to type 1 herpes affords a very high degree of protection against infection with type 2 herpes. This protection makes type 2 somewhat more difficult to get. Antibody to type 1 herpes, however, does not *fully* protect against type 2. Many people who get type 2 herpes do so despite having this type 1 partial protection. People with type 1 who do get type 2 will, by definition, not experience a true primary. The first episode will likely be less severe than for people who have no preexisting immunity to type 1 or type 2. It may be that people with type 1 immunity are somewhat predisposed to acquire type 2 genital herpes asymptomatically, should they come in contact with type 2 herpes and acquire infection from a partner. Since their bodies are already fully equipped to fight off the infection effectively, people with type 1 herpes are probably more likely not to notice infection with type 2. Type 1 herpes is just as likely as type 2 herpes, however, to be acquired without any evident symptoms-so, while a history of recurrent oral cold sores is strongly suggestive of type 1 herpes simplex, the absence of such a history provides absolutely no evidence that a person does not have latent herpes simplex virus type 1. Only typespecific antibody tests like the Western blot are able to do that.

How could this happen to me?

Herpes infection can happen to anyone. Several careful epidemiological studies have proven this. Approximately four out of five people with genital herpes acquire their genital herpes infection some time between their eighteenth and thirty-sixth birthdays. The overall incidence of genital herpes (apparent and unapparent) is increasing constantly. Most genital herpes infections are unknown to the people who have them (asymptomatic or unapparent). The group of people at greatest risk are women between the ages of twenty and twenty-four. Depending upon the group being studied, approximately 16 to 33 percent of Americans have antibody to type 2 herpes simplex virus. In other words, those people actually have type 2 genital herpes, even though most of them do not recognize that fact. On a statistical basis, the more sexual partners a person has had, the more likely that he or she will have antibody to type 2 herpes. In all age groups, African-Americans have been shown to be at greater risk of having antibody to type 2 herpes than Caucasians of the same age. Australians have about half to two-thirds the incidence of type 2 herpes compared with North Americans. Observations regarding income of people with herpes have been somewhat inconsistent. In many studies, antibody to type 2 herpes is more prevalent in people of lower income. However, in one Stanford study, Hispanic women who were of upper middle class income were far more likely than lower income women to be seropositive for type 2 herpes (30 percent versus 17 percent). Studies from herpes self-help groups also show very high levels of education and income among people diagnosed with herpes. I am sure that it is not the college or the job that gave that person genital herpes. Nor is herpes caused by a specific race or socioeconomic class.

Herpes literally knows no boundaries. Even sexual habits may not correlate in anyone individual to the acquisition of infection. You only need to have one lifetime sexual partner to get genital herpes. Even if both you and your partner have only been with each other in your whole lives, it is quite possible for you to get type 1 genital herpes from oral-genital sexual contact if your partner has mouth infection. If your partner has had previous sexual partners even a long time ago, there is a good chance that he or she has come across this infection. If your partner has had more than ten sexual partners in the past, he or she is statistically likely to have been infected with herpes. By statistical chances alone, people with more sexual contacts are more likely to acquire this virus. There is an additional approximately 5 to 6 percent risk for each additional sexual partner. However, herpes has become so universal that many people who have had only one or two sexual contacts have herpes. Since genital herpes is predominantly an external disease, sexual contact that results in transmission does not necessarily include vaginal penetration. Several well-documented cases of herpes in women who have not had vaginal intercourse have been described, almost always the result of oral-genital contact.

As a society, we have subjected ourselves to a higher chance of running into herpes, partly by giving up condoms and foam for the convenience of the intrauterine device QUO) and the pill and partly because sex has become less forbidden. Oral sex has become

104

commonplace, while oral-to-oral transmission of type 1 herpes simplex virus in childhood has become less likely. These factors lead to an increase in oral-to-genital transmission of herpes. Herpes infection of some type is found in most people on earth. Sores on the genitals usually come with more emotional baggage than sores on the mouth. But the stigma attached to genital herpes is mainly a media phenomenon. Genital herpes is basically a nuisance skin infection that comes and goes. It has unusual complications that are unlikely to occur and are highly preventable.

Some people have suggested that the growing incidence of herpes is a new demonstration of the wrath of God. In response to this, I would point out that elimination of all but monogamous sexual contact would cut down the overall incidence of this infection, but monogamy would not eliminate herpes. A person who was monogamous or even sexually inactive could get genital herpes. Increasing the numbers of sexual partners statistically increases the chances of getting any sexually transmitted disease. For the sake of prevention of disease, it is and always has been wise to be selective, to know your partner, to avoid casual sex, etc. Religious preference does not correlate in any way to susceptibility to infection, however. Herpes is no more a sign of punishment from God than Legionnaire's disease was a sign of punishment from God inflicted upon the American Legion. Ascribing any new disease or affliction, or any old disease or affliction, to the plagues of God is rewriting the Bible. In the case of herpes, it is also the result of misinformation.

I had sex last night and awoke with a sore. Did I spread herpes to my partner? Should my partner be taking an oral antiviral drug to prevent infection?

Probably not, if you had no symptoms of active infection when you had genital contact. Herpes shedding does not generally begin before the symptoms of an outbreak, although studies done at the University of Washington did show that shedding of virus just before the onset of genital symptoms was the probable source of asymptomatic transmission in several cases. In some cases, a recurrent herpes sore will start out as an asymptomatic episode, probably because the sore is too small or mild to detect. For whatever reason, it goes unnoticed. Then, by the next day, the sore is bigger or more swollen or more uncomfortable-in other words, more symptomatic. This is not the normal situation, but it is apparently not rare either. To awaken with a sore without having had or having noticed a prodrome is a relatively frequent event that is usually, although not always, a new event, totally unconnected to the asymptomatic day or night before.

Furthermore, if sexual contact is a daily occurrence, then every time you awake with herpes you will have had sex the night before. If you have followed the guidelines for preventing transmission, including use of safer sex practices, then even if you had a small sore that went unnoticed, your partner will have been protected by those just-in-case efforts. However, if you think that you may have exposed your partner to direct contact with an active sore, then your partner may wish to consider using one of the oral antiviral drugs, because even though this type of treatment is unproven for this purpose, there is every reason to believe that it could provide some protection following exposure in some people (see chapter 11). This is not a method to count on, however. As a side note, there is no scientific justification for a susceptible partner to take antiviral medications on a long-term or continuing basis. Preventive use for one week after a likely exposure is also unproven but makes some sense based on research in animals and on the high degree of safety seen with these medicines. Long-term use by someone who does not have herpes at all would be quite another matter. For further information, refer to chapter 11.

Can I have a long-term relationship with one person and never transmit herpes?

Yes, such relationships are very common. Dr. Charles Prober at Stanford University has found that couples are very commonly "discordant"-that is, one person has type 2 genital herpes-without transmitting it to the partner, often for a very long time.

In general, the chance of not seeing an active sore becomes higher as the number of encounters between two people increases. It is often the case, however, that when herpes is transmitted after a

couple has been together for several years with only one partner affected, there has been an event during which the barrier to active infection broke down. A break in the barrier to active infection can occur because of a mistake, because of a choice, or because of asymptomatic virus shedding.

In time, many couples lose their desire to hold to strict rules to avoid transmission. Since herpes is usually physically mild, some people in permanent relationships decide that prevention is not worthwhile. Once the issue of discussing herpes with your partner has been dealt with and the relationship has established itself as long-term, couples often choose to ignore the small ongoing risk of transmission and begin taking risks.

Speaking of risks, we take them all the time. We risk our lives driving in cars; we risk our genital health having sex. To take risks is human. To take risks with someone with herpes is also human and, relative to some other risks, not so big. Deciding which risks are right for you is up to each individual and each couple.

Herpes of the Newborn

What is herpes of the newborn?

Despite dramatic breakthroughs in knowledge, our understanding of immunology (the body's defense network) leaves a lot unexplained. The immunology of the newborn baby is especially confusing. At birth, many changes take place. The heart begins pumping blood in a different direction, the lungs inflate with air for the first time, and the baby becomes a free-living organism facing the external environment. Most babies thrive in this new environment. For reasons that are only partially understood, some babies are highly susceptible to infection.

Many different infectious agents cause infections in newborns under certain circumstances. Most of these agents are entirely tolerable to adults. They may even be normal flora-a part of the normal (indeed, necessary) colony of bacteria or fungi that cause absolutely no disease in adults. One example of normal flora is the bacteria *Escherichia coli,* which inhabits the gut of nearly everyone. Commonly, a woman gets some of these bacteria into her bladder-often as a consequence of minor trauma from sexual contact-and a urinary tract infection (cystitis) results.

Most babies tolerate this organism. Essentially all babies are exposed to it during birth. Of 1,000 babies who are exposed, 998 could not care less. However, an unfortunate one or two of the thousand develop severe, overwhelming infection-even meningitis-and may suffer severe damage or even die. In some of these babies, the reason for infection is obvious-for example, prolonged rupture of the membranes, where exposure to bacteria may be very intense and sustained over a long period. In other cases, the reasons for infection remain unknown.

Why should a newborn baby be so susceptible to infection?

Every baby's immune system is somewhat immature. Immune experience is nearly as undeveloped as job experience at birth, except that the mother's blood gives some immune experience to the baby by passing along antibodies, which filter across the placenta. Newborns are born possessing many of the same antibodies as their mothers. While inside the uterus, the fetus is protected from most infection by the filtering capabilities of the placenta, which excludes almost all infecting agents; at the time of birth, the newborn has not yet had to respond to infection. All those lymphocytes and macrophages and so forth, which do most of the immune fighting against foreign invaders, have never been stimulated before. Just as the newborn has never before seen the light of day, so her or his white blood cells have never seen a bacterium. The cells are just beginning to learn how the system works. Thus, occasionally, a baby succumbs to an infection that would cause only a mild illness or no problem at all in you or me.

Herpes of the newborn is one example of this problem. Herpes simplex, which causes a mild skin infection in the adult, may, under certain circumstances, overcome the immature immune system of a newborn baby and disseminate throughout the body, resulting in death, or ascend up the immature nervous system into the brain, resulting in encephalitis with consequent brain damage, or invade the eye, resulting in eye infection and eye damage. Such complications are very unlikely to occur in any individual newborn. All studies in the past decade have shown that herpes simplex infection is extremely unlikely to occur to anyone individual baby born to a woman with genital herpes. In fact, the woman's infection with herpes before pregnancy even offers some protection to the baby if exposure to active herpes takes place. Curiously, more than half the babies born with herpes have mothers who did not know they had herpes. If a pregnant woman knows she has genital herpes, newborn herpes is largely preventable and highly unlikely. Herpes is not a reason to avoid having children, because the baby of a woman with genital herpes is extremely unlikely to have any problems with neonatal (newborn) infection.

What are the signs?

Just as the symptoms of genital herpes vary with the location of the infection, so do the signs of neonatal herpes. In some unusual cases, herpes is already present at birth. Since infection usually begins at the time of birth, however, it most commonly takes several days to a couple of weeks to become evident. The most common herpes infection in newborns is on the skin. The skin sore looks much like a sore on an adult-Le., a single vesicle (blister) or cluster of vesicles. Occasionally, herpes begins as a red or purplish rash. Because many very mild skin rashes of infancy mimic herpes, it is important to ask a doctor's opinion when a skin rash develops in a newborn-especially if a sore similar to those pictured in chapter 3 develops. Almost every baby has some type of skin rash at some point in the first few weeks of life. Normal things called *milia,* for example, which look like little pimples, may be frightening to the mother with genital herpes who thinks her baby has the infection. Milia are very, very common; several babies in every nursery have them. Expect to see a skin rash on your baby just because he or she is a baby. Genuine herpes sores may be found anywhere on the skin, especially on the head of a baby born head first, the buttocks of a baby born rear first, and so on. Plate 13 (page 101) shows a newborn who was delivered feet first. Skin lesions in a newborn are not always or exclusively at the site of the presenting part, however. Plate 14 (page 101) shows the recurrent herpes on the hand of a baby that had neonatal herpes at birth.

Another common site of herpes of the newborn is the eyes.
Most babies have red and swollen eyes because of the silver nitrate put in their eyes at birth to prevent infection. Generally, the redness and discharge fades Quickly over the first few days of life. Herpes in the eye most often appears as *redness-conjunc-*

110

tivitis-with or without discharge of pus from the eye. Herpes infection of the eye is often detectable only by an examination by an ophthalmologist (eye specialist).

Most studies suggest that many newborns who develop genital herpes never develop skin lesions at all. The more severe neonatal herpes syndromes are infection of the central nervous system (the brain) and infection that disseminates through being carried in the blood and distributed in many parts of the body. Brain infection tends to appear at one to four weeks of age. An affected baby may suddenly lose his or her active behavior and become lethargic. The baby may stop caring about things such as feeding, or may do just the opposite and become very irritable. This, of course, is a very common thing in normal babies as well, but an irritable baby should be assessed to make sure it is nothing more than "just colic." Shaking, twitching, or fits (like epileptic fits) should be checked out by a physician without delay. Babies with herpes infection of the nervous system may have skin sores, but very often a baby with serious herpes infection shows no skin problem whatsoever.

The same is true for disseminated herpes; skin sores mayor may not be present. Dissemination appears a bit earlier, often within the first seven days of life. In most cases, herpes is present at birth, implying that herpes infected the baby inside the womb. There is no known specific method for prevention of womb infection. Most babies with dissemination have nonspecific symptoms, including lethargy, going off feeding, and vomiting. An affected baby may become gravely ill very rapidly. *Jaundice* (yellow skin) is very common in infants. When associated with actual liver enlargement and abnormal blood tests of liver function, jaundice may be the result of herpes or it may be caused by many other things. Sometimes a baby with herpes gets *pneumonia,* has difficulty breathing, or has *apnea* (spells with no breathing at all). These are serious problems that require intensive investigation in hospital. If the mother has herpes, the pediatrician needs to know in order to consider this possibility.

All of the scenarios discussed above, with the possible exception of skin sores, have nonspecific symptoms. This is the problem. So many things-some infectious, some noninfectious; some very serious, some very minor-present themselves in exactly the same way. Reading this section may be frightening, but reading the list of symptoms of any disease can be frightening. Even if your baby gets all of these symptoms, herpes is unlikely. Neonatal herpes is exceedingly unlikely to occur and is highly preventable. Furthermore, if it happens in spite of efforts at prevention, it is treatable. In fact, the problem with treatment is less the difficulty of finding a useful drug and more the delay that often occurs before the diagnosis is made. If the first sign of something serious is nonspecific, it may take days to find the correct diagnosis. The delay makes treatment more difficult. If your infant becomes ill, get medical attention. Herpes can be diagnosed only if it is looked for; tell your physician about your herpes to make sure he or she considers herpes as a possibility. You should not attempt to make your own diagnosis.

Is direct contact during delivery the only way of giving herpes to a baby?

No, but it is by far the most common way of transmitting it. Most often, newborn herpes infection results from a lack of awareness by everyone concerned. Most people (includingpregnant women) with herpes never know that they have herpes. Once recurrent herpes has occurred, nature takes over and, by a series of brilliant maneuvers, effectively prevent herpes transmission to the newborn in the vast majority of potential cases. Once recurrent herpes has been diagnosed, the woman and her health care provider can do many more things to prevent transmission. We are learning, however, that we have to be careful in trying to improve on the prevention techniques of nature, because some of our previously accepted prevention techniques have proven to be worse for the mother than the very low risk of neonatal herpes ever was. Babies of women with recurrent genital herpes are largely protected from infection with herpes, for reasons described later in this chapter.

When herpes is not diagnosed before the woman gives birth, however, prevention is left entirely up to nature. In the case of recurrent herpes, the baby may be exposed to active virus on the mother's skin. This does not lead to any problem in the newborn in the vast majority of cases, but physicians generally believe that if exposure to known virus on the skin in an active phase of infection can be prevented during labor and delivery, it should be. In other words, someone who is having an active recurrence should have a cesarean section. There is argument about this, too, however, since there is a small but significant risk of complications from cesarean section. In most cases, a baby born to a mother having an active herpes episode will not develop any disease as a result of this exposure, so we should be very careful in trying to improve on this already impressive capability of nature.

The situation is different, however, if a woman develops primary herpes or nonprimary type 2 herpes (first time ever in a patient who has never been previously exposed) during the last few days or weeks of pregnancy. It is common for first episodes of infection to begin with nonspecific symptoms-for example, vaginal discharge, fever, or urinary discomfort. There may not be obvious external sores early on. The woman experiencing a first episode may very well not realize what is going on and therefore not warn her physician. Furthermore, a visual search for herpes may not be done during labor and delivery. The exam for herpes is a visual one and includes a search for uncomfortable sores on the vaginal lips, on the perineum, around the anus, under the pubic hair, and on the cervix. The usual obstetric exam during labor, however, is a manual one-a search for the progress of labor, using the fingers to feel the cervix. Feeling with the fingers does not detect herpes sores. The eyes detect herpes. Newborns of mothers having a first episode herpes infection are likely to be undiagnosed and are also especially susceptible to getting herpes.

So what should be done to prevent transmission of herpes to the newborn? People must learn to think about herpes when vaginal discomfort or other symptoms appear during the latter part of pregnancy. Physicians who deliver babies must make their eyes an important part of their medical tool kits during labor. Every woman in labor, regardless of her history, should be assessed for herpes by careful examination. Some hospitals have begun to assess each woman by virus culture as well, but, because results take one to several days to be returned, viral culture cannot be used to determine whether cesarean section is necessary. If active genital herpes is visible near the birth canal, cesarean section is probably advised, even for a woman with recurrent genital herpes. However, if no lesion is present, the very low risk of transmission of herpes does not warrant the use of cesarean section for the prevention of herpes. In contrast, where a first episode (primary or nonprimary) of genital herpes occurs in the late second or third trimester of pregnancy, neonatal herpes risk can be greater. In such situations, some specialists would recommend treatment with acyclovir for ten days, even though no studies have been performed and no clear guidelines are available. Some (but not all) would restart acyclovir for the last four weeks of pregnancy. For now, this is an individual decision and must be made between the woman and her physician.

Neonatal herpes can occasionally be caused by infection after birth. These cases are relatively unusual. Since the mother may not even have herpes, there is a high chance that the baby will be born without immunity from the mother and be very susceptible. Exposure can come, for example, from the kiss of a parent or nursery attendant who has an active cold sore. The *herpetic whitlow* (herpes of the finger) is an especially important cause for concern, since this infection is often misdiagnosed (see figure 11, page 199). Because the herpes is on the finger, any finger-to-skin contact from the affected person when whitlows are active could result in transmission of herpes. Also, if another baby in the nursery has herpes, a nurse who handles the infected baby and does not wash his or her hands might pass on the virus to another infant. Happily, hospitals have strong infection control measures to prevent this.

Infection can also occur inside the womb, although this occurs rarely. Probably most fetuses infected with herpes early in gestation (their time inside the womb) do not survive and are miscarried. Because infection with herpes can be spotty, however, it is possible for infection to occur at one area that is not crucial to survival and for the fetus to develop in spite of this infection. Near term, it is possible (though unlikely) for little holes in the amnion (sac of waters) to open and reseal, allowing infection in. Fortunately, this is unlikely to lead to herpes infection. Herpes infection in the newborn generally occurs during birth. The congenital (inside the womb) herpes syndrome does exist, however, and there is nothing that can be done specifically to prevent it. It cannot be predicted on the basis of the type of infection or by special tests. There is no greater risk in babies whose mothers have five outbreaks per month than in those whose mothers have one outbreak per year. In fact, why it ever happens is poorly understood. Some cases result from true primary herpes during pregnancy.

Can I transmit herpes by kissing my baby?

Yes, as described above. Neonatal herpes can be type 1 or type 2. Approximately one-fourth of neonatal infections are type 1. It is not actually *proven* that kissing is an important source for neonatal herpes. It is likely that type 1 neonatal herpes often results from the mother's primary genital type 1 infection. It is prudent to assume that kissing and other nongenital contact can also cause neonatal herpes, despite academic argument to the contrary. A kiss from a herpes-infected mouth can transmit herpes as well as a delivery through a herpes-infected vagina. If you have sores on your mouth just after the baby is born, transmission must be carefully avoided. (Of course, people with genital herpes do not have to avoid kissing newborns. Genital herpes cannot jump from your genitals to your mouth to your baby.)

What is done to prevent transmission after birth? First, if herpes is not active in the mother, nothing special is done. Birth proceeds normally and the baby is treated exactly like any other baby. He or she may room in, or stay in the nursery, or both. Whatever you want to arrange with the doctor and the hospital is just fine. If herpes is *active* on the genitals when labor begins, a cesarean section is performed (more on that later), and the baby should usually room in with the mother or be in a special area of the nursery. Otherwise, things are routine. You need not wear a mask unless you have a sore on your mouth. You need not wear gloves unless you have a sore your hands. You can breast-feed without problems unless you have a sore on your breast. You should not find yourself in strict isolation in the hospital because of herpes. You might find an isolation sign on your door saying "Contact Isolation" or "Wound and Skin Isolation", meaning that your sore, if active, should be isolated while you are in the hospital. Nothing else need be isolated. Most precautions in hospitals make sense. Someone should be able to explain why you and your baby need or do not need to be isolated. There should be neither too little nor too much isolation. If your questions are not properly answered, you might ask to speak with the infection control officer (usually a nurse or physician) for an explanation.

Why does first episode primary or nonprimary type 2 herpes during pregnancy pose a much greater risk for the newborn?

Primary herpes affects the mother's whole body. Illness in the mother can cause early labor and premature birth, a significant risk factor for developing neonatal herpes. Primary herpes occurs, by definition, before the mother has acquired any immunity to herpes. Nonprimary type 2 first episodes of herpes occur before the mother has acquired any immunity to that virus. As the mother has no immunity to pass on to the baby, the baby is born susceptible to herpes infection. Furthermore, because primary herpes in most cases involves the internal parts of the birth canal, including the cervix, exposure of the newborn is much more likely to occur. First episodes of herpes are very likely to go undiagnosed because the symptoms are often nonspecific and the diagnosis unsuspected. In addition, the amount of virus shedding is very high compared with a recurrent episode-as much as a thousand times more. Viral shedding tends to last for ten to fourteen days, rather than two or three days in a recurrent episode.

What if my partner has genital herpes and J do not?

Some studies have suggested that we may be better able to prevent neonatal herpes in the future by focusing more on undiagnosed cases of maternal primary infection. The best way to prevent primary or nonprimary type 2 herpes infections in pregnant women is to prevent exposure to herpes during pregnancy. One logical way to do this is to identify situations where the pregnant woman's sexual partner has genital herpes and the pregnant woman does not. Dr. Charles Prober and his colleagues at Stanford University have begun to study the possibility of identifying such *discordant pairs,* in which the partner has herpes and the pregnant woman does not. That combination has the potential for a bad outcome. People who have herpes should discuss this with their partners if pregnancy is planned. The pregnant woman who has never had herpes and who continues to have sexual contact with a partner with herpes is in a powder keg situation, as far as neonatal herpes is concerned. It is important that she not acquire infection for the first time during pregnancy, especially toward the last trimester. If she gets herpes before pregnancy, then the baby is at low risk because of the reasons given elsewhere in this chapter. If she gets herpes after pregnancy, the baby is not, of course, at risk. However if she gets herpes for the first time during pregnancy, the baby's risk is significant. Accurate determination of her susceptibility requires the type-specific blood test, as outlined in chapter 4. Couples who have given up safer sexual practices should readopt them during pregnancy if the pregnant woman remains susceptible to herpes. Safer sex in this case means avoiding genital sexual contact altogether during active phases of infection and using the prevention techniques described in chapter 12 when having sexual contact at inactive times. The couple should take every possible measure to prevent transmission of herpes during the pregnancy.

Preventing transmission of herpes during pregnancy will be one of the most important challenges for any new herpes vaccine. You can read more about vaccines in chapter 11.

If a pregnant woman does acquire true primary genital herpes, I advise the following:

1. Document the infection, using viral culture of the lesions.

2. Rule out other sexually transmitted diseases and the common vaginal infection bacterial vaginosis, since they can also have special impact during pregnancy, if left untreated.

3. Determine whether it is a primary or nonprimary type 2 herpes infection. This is possible in most cases by determining that the initial serology (Western blot) test for herpes is totally negative (true primary) or negative for type 2 and positive for type 1 (nonprimary), meaning that the person is susceptible. If this negative test is combined with a positive viral test for herpes

from the genital tract, the diagnosis of a true primary or a nonprimary genital herpes infection is confirmed.

4. If a primary is suspected during a first episode, because of severe lesions on both sides of the body, fever, cervical involvement, inguinal lymph node (gland) swelling and tenderness, or urinary symptoms, or, if a possible primary infection is documented (as discussed above), then systemic treatment with acyclovir may be warranted, despite the fact that the safety of acyclovir during pregnancy is not fully proven (see below).

5. In some situations, your doctor may decide with you to prescribe oral acyclovir for treating your first episode. However, this is an individual clinical decision between you and your doctor, since no scientific studies are available to provide guidelines.

6. You and your doctor should discuss the option of cesarean section if your primary or nonprimary first episode of genital herpes infection took place during the third trimester of pregnancy, regardless of the clinical state of your herpes at the time of labor. This is not a proven approach and has not been discussed much in the medical literature. However, the risk of having a positive cervical culture in the absence of any symptoms is higher than usual during the first three months after the primary. This risk, which is much higher than the risk of asymptomatic shedding during any later asymptomatic phase of genital herpes, may warrant planned cesarean section (at term) for a woman who has had a first genital infection in the third trimester. Cesarean section for asymptomatic herpes is not warranted in any situation other than the true primary or nonprimary first episode in the third trimester, however, for reasons outlined elsewhere in this chapter.

Why am I advised to avoid acyclovir during pregnancy, on the one hand, and to use acyclovir during pregnancy, on the other hand?

There is every reason to believe that the use of acyclovir during pregnancy is *probably* safe. Probably safe is not good enough, of course, to warrant the use of this drug for trivial reasons. Therefore, in most cases where it does not matter, acyclovir should be discontinued during pregnancy. This is especially important during early pregnancy, when the risk of harm to the fetus is greatest. In the third trimester, the fetus has formed most of its key organs already. Acyclovir does not *seem* harmful, so far, even where it has been used in early pregnancy. Studies have shown that untreated primary herpes in the third trimester may result in a significant medical problem for the newborn in up to 50 percent of cases. Therefore, intervention with treatment is very logical. Treatment of the pregnant woman with acyclovir, however, has not been fully *proven* to be safe or effective. Although there is no scientific evidence, it is possible that there could be a benefit to the woman and the fetus by reducing the severity of primary herpes, including the viral load and the duration of complications, which could theoretically reduce the chance of the baby developing a medical problem.

This opinion is guesswork, though, in the absence of a study.

Some doctors and scientists argue that it is better to let the mother acquire the best possible immunity to the virus on her own. Treatment with acyclovir probably limits the degree of immunity the mother acquires, by limiting the amount of time and the degree to which she is exposed to the virus in order to develop immunity to it. In theory, that could wind up being worse for the baby than no treatment at all. I believe it is important to limit the severity of the primary episode, if at all possible. But this course of action is unproven and should be decided in each individual case by the woman and her doctor. No one simple answer is available now, and the chance of a definitive clinical trial is minimal. Chances are we will continue to do what we think best. The more acyclovir's safety record suggests that it is free of significant harm in pregnancy, the better this approach appears.

What about the newer antiviral drugs, tamciclooir and oalacyclooir?
Both are probably safe in pregnancy, but because there is far less clinical experience with new drugs, acyclovir should probably be the main drug to consider when using a drug in pregnancy. You

will have to make this decision with your doctor, however, and he or she is the best source for up-to-date information about risks and benefits.

If I get primary herpes during early pregnancy, should I have an abortion?

If herpes were ever to spread into the womb, it would be most likly to occur during primary herpes, before immunity to the virus is established. If a fetus were to be infected with herpes early in gestation, the likelihood of miscarriage would probably be very high. A recent study by Dr. Z. A. Brown from the University of Washington described the outcome of fifteen cases of primary genital herpes during pregnancy. One of the five fetuses of women affected during the first trimester (twelve weeks) was spontaneously miscarried and had been infected in the womb with herpes. The other four were fine. Subsequent studies by Brown have suggested that the actual risk to the fetus of primary infection in the first trimester may be much smaller than the small initial studies suggested. But more work needs to be done.

Is herpes, then, an indication for therapeutic abortion? A lot will depend on the woman's attitude toward abortion and toward the pregnancy. Even if a woman is in her eighth week and having fullblown primary herpes, her fetus's risk of becoming infected in the womb is low. Exactly how low remains to be determined. The woman must decide what to do. By no stretch of the imagination is genital herpes a necessary reason to have an abortion.

In order to make any decision about a possible abortion, or any other course of action, you must first be certain you have your facts straight. Recurrent herpes and nonprimary first episodes are not reasons for abortion, so you should be quite certain first that what you had was a true primary. Clinical differences between true primary and non primary first episodes are often blurred and may be misleading-especially in pregnancy. The diagnosis should be unequivocal. This means determining that the following are true:

1. It was your first ever vaginal sore like this;

2. A herpes culture test was positive;

3. In association with a positive herpes culture, a herpes antibody test was negative at the outset of the infection; and/or

4. Your physician feels that your symptoms were typical of primary herpes (many sores involving both sides of the genitals, lasting longer than ten days, and often associated with swollen inguinal nodes or "glands" or fever and headache).

In general, you should not have amniocentesis to find out anything about herpes. Amniocentesis can be very informative for other reasons, but amniocentesis for herpes can be misleading. Look for answers about herpes in other ways, as described above.

What can I do to prevent my baby from contracting my herpes? Discuss herpes with your doctor early in your pregnancy. An ultrasound study early in pregnancy might be useful for determining dates. If and when the time comes for deciding whether a cesarean section is necessary, it is easiest if the doctor has all the available facts concerning when the baby is really due.

Learn the active phases of infection, monitor yourself for herpes, and report recurrences to your doctor.

If you have a symptomatic active recurrence during the last four to six weeks of pregnancy, see your doctor as soon as you can after the start of the recurrence. He or she should assess the sore and perform a culture to confirm what it is. As soon as the sore is healed, the area should be cultured again so that there is laboratory proof that the area is virus-free before you elect to have a normal vaginal birth. Guidelines from the American College of Obstetrics and Gynecology Committee recommend that every woman with a history of genital herpes have at least one negative culture before labor (with no subsequent new symptoms of active herpes) before deciding on the normal route of delivery. Yet doing weekly cultures near term without symptoms seemed to be a poor method of prevention of infection in one study in California. Studies have proven that neonatal herpes is extremely unlikely to occur, even if the mother with recurrent herpes is culture-positive during labor! The best way to prevent neonatal herpes, therefore, is an area of continuing academic controversy. I recommend that your doctor carefully examine with a strong light source the external genitals (shown in figure 6b, page 50) on your last two or three prenatal visits and once again during labor. This will let your doctor know what your genital skin normally looks like, so that he or she will be fairly confident that the appearance is normal during labor before electing to assist with a vaginal birth. A virus culture, using one moistened swab of all of the external genital areas, should be taken on at least one of the prenatal visits and repeated during labor. If a sore or symptoms of a sore are present at labor, a cesarean section is indicated. If all looks well, and the last virus culture is negative, a cesarean is not required.

Unless there is a very important reason for using one, a fetal scalp monitor should probably be avoided if you have a history of herpes.

Obtain a cesarean section if and only if you have *active* herpes or you have just had active herpes that your doctor thinks might not be healed when you go into labor. The decision about whether herpes is healed can be a tough one. Essentially we are considering the active phases (chapter 3) as active and the inactive as inactive. A culture is especially useful in keeping the time to a minimum. If the episode near the end of term is a *primary* one, it would be wise to extend the safety period because of the high risk of asymptomatic viral shedding following primary infection. I tend to use systemic acyclovir to treat primary herpes in late pregnancy and continue to use acyclovir for suppression of herpes until delivery. Because the risk of asymptomatic shedding on the cervix is very high during the few months following a first episode of genital herpes, I recommend cesarean section for most cases of true primary or non primary type 2 herpes infection during the third trimester.

If your herpes is active, a cesarean section is urgently needed once membranes rupture. The operation can be arranged less urgently after the onset of labor if the membranes are intact. If herpes is not active, a cesarean is not necessary.

Does a cesarean delivery always prevent transmission? Because herpes is generally transmitted by direct contact, when a physical barrier (the bag of waters) remains between a herpes sore and a baby's skin, the risk of neonatal infection is extremely small. Thus, bypassing an active sore by delivering the baby through the abdomen (cesarean section) is an extremely effective method of prevention. Whether or not you will need a cesarean section depends on whether you are in an active phase of infection when labor begins. The statistical likelihood of needing a cesarean section will depend on how often you get recurrences. As far as we know, a high recurrence frequency rate will not detrimentally affect the risk to your baby. First episode genital infection during pregnancy, especially late pregnancy, is a different matter and is discussed elsewhere in this chapter.

Once the sac of waters is broken, the possibility of direct transmission to the baby becomes more likely. If this occurs without your knowing it (there may be small holes that heal up without symptoms), then a cesarean section may not prevent infection. The practical risk of membranes rupturing without your knowledge and causing problems is very small, however.

Confusion might arise in identifying when the bag of waters breaks; leaky fluid is usually obvious, but sudden clear fluid discharges in late pregnancy need checking out at a hospital. Once the membranes rupture-and this may be the first symptom of laborit is only a matter of time until active herpes on the outside gets to the inside. This is because the barrier is broken and a wet path has developed. In other words, there is a fluid connection from outside to inside held nicely at body temperature, allowing the virus to find its way inside. If herpes is active on the skin when the membranes rupture, it is only a matter of time before the virus gets to the baby. Therefore, cesarean section has to be done immediately. There has been some discussion recently suggesting that it is all right to wait four hours from the time membranes rupture until the cesarean section is performed. This is not true. If herpes is considered to be active at the time the membranes rupture, a cesarean section should be performed as soon as possible.

If recurrent herpes is active and membranes have not been ruptured for a prolonged period of time, cesarean section is often the best way of helping the body in the job it is already performing of efficiently and effectively preventing herpes transmission to the newborn. Arguments are being made by health economists and statisticians and even some clinical experts, however, that would suggest holding back with cesarean section except in cases of true primary or non primary type 2 genital infection. For now, I prefer to stick with the long-practiced approach of recommending cesarean section if there is evidence of an active episode of recurrent herpes. Chances are, though, that the newborn baby will be healthy regardless of which path the woman with recurrent herpes and her doctor choose. First episodes of genital herpes during late pregnancy are a different matter and need specialized care.

Why don't all pregnant women with genital herpes have cesarean sections?

Some pregnant women with herpes feel that cesarean is the way to go regardless of the situation. Often this stems from the burden of guilt that the woman feels would arise from an infection in the baby. This is a very noble thought indeed, but it is often based on a lack of understanding of the facts. Here are the facts:

1. Genital herpes is a common problem, while neonatal herpes is an uncommon one.

2. A cesarean section may be needed if herpes is active during labor. Even in those cases of recurrent herpes where we have traditionally considered cesarean section necessary, however, medical experts and epidemiologists are beginning to question this approach. While it still remains the current standard of medical practice to recommend cesarean section during an active genital recurrence, there is little proof that this approach significantly improves the natural protection conferred by the woman's own immunity and the limited lesion area exposure found during a mild recurrence. If we are beginning to question the validity of cesarean section during an active episode, it makes even less sense to opt for cesarean section when herpes is inactive. With the exception of the post-first episode, if episodes of recurrent genital herpes are not active during labor, cesarean section offers no advantages over normal vaginal birth.

3. Despite its overall good safety record, the risk of cesarean section to the mother is much higher than that of vaginal birth.

After all, cesarean birth is a form of surgery. It means a longer hospital stay and a higher risk of postpartum (after birth) complications to the mother, such as fever and infection. The risk of cesarean section is low, but the risks of surgery clearly outweigh any potential benefits when herpes is not active at the time of labor.

4. Even cesarean section won't necessarily prevent neonatal herpes, which can come from other sources than the mother's genital herpes-for example, transmission of herpes from Aunt Sadie's fever blister. It is much better to think out the problem and use care in avoiding transmission. A prevention panacea may just obscure the issues.

If acyclovir is probably safe during pregnancy, why can't I take it to prevent the need for cesarean section?

This technique is under study, and initial data suggest that this may be a very effective approach. (Antiviral treatment in general is further discussed in chapter 11.) The official stand is that treatment is not advised until further studies show that this approach is safe and effective. To date, the studies performed have not been large enough to draw complete conclusions. As discussed earlier in this chapter, oral acyclovir is probably safe in pregnancy. Since the indication for cesarean section is the appearance of a clinical recurrence of herpes during labor, and since acyclovir suppression has been shown to reduce the rates of clinical recurrence dramatically, it follows that acyclovir suppression would markedly reduce the number of cesarean sections performed for herpes recurrences. If no harm came to the mother or baby, then this cost-effective use of medication would be of great benefit, since it would limit the duration of hospitalization and complications from the cesarean sections done for herpes. It will be virtually impossible to prove that this suppressive approach is effective at reducing the rate of neonatal herpes, since in most cases mothers with first episode genital herpes infection are not undergoing any drug intervention or serial assessment. There just aren't enough cases to show that any treatment would prevent disease in the baby.

There are several possible negative aspects to acyclovir treatment during late pregnancy:

1. This treatment has not been proven safe in pregnancy. It is possible that some hidden side effects of treatment in pregnancy will emerge later. There are theoretical concerns that kidney damage or reduced white blood cell counts in the newborn might occur.

2. There is no evidence to favor the idea that taking acyclovir might protect the baby from getting herpes. It would be used, instead, to improve the likelihood of the pregnant woman having a vaginal delivery. Thus, there is no guarantee that the use of acyclovir (or any other drug) will prevent newborns from getting herpes.

3. Neonatal herpes occurred in one baby in a study where acyclovir suppression was used for this purpose.

4. It is possible that suppression with acyclovir could mask a recurrence without fully preventing viral shedding. It is thus theoretically possible that acyclovir treatment might actually increase the chance of missing an active episode and exposing the baby to active virus.

Despite these possible negatives, there are a lot of potential positives that warrant consideration of this approach. Probably the strongest positive reason suggesting that acyclovir suppression may be sensible in late pregnancy is its positive effect on reducing asymptomatic viral shedding. But until definitive data prove the correct approach, I believe that the potential benefit could be very good, assuming that definitive clinical trials support some of the preliminary information suggesting that this approach may reduce the cesarean section rate. Unfortunately, the safety of this treatment is unproven. Therefore, if a pregnant woman wishes, and if she understands that this is not a proven area, and especially if she has high recurrence frequency rates that are very likely to require her to have a cesarean section, I would proceed carefully, using 1,000 to 1,200 mg per day in three to six doses. I would still recommend cesarean section for an active episode, and I would still like to see the mother cultured during labor and the baby cultured after birth for herpes to be sure nothing was missed. Whenever a drug is used outside of the list of possible indications from the FDA (or its equivalent in your country) it becomes an area of hot controversy. On the one hand, physicians and patients need to be able to proceed on the basis of best clinical judgment in areas where treatment is likely to work. On the other hand, we do not know with certainty that the treatment as described in this chapter is effective. Sometimes expensive, ineffective, or even harmful treatments get entrenched without proof into common clinical practice. For now, there is the clear possibility that treatment could turn out to be worse than no treatment. On the other hand, to miss the chance at having a normal vaginal birth while waiting for the data to become available is also a potential unnecessary loss. Discuss the issues with your doctor. Do not take it upon yourself, under any circumstances, to use acyclovir during pregnancy or otherwise, without the prescription of your doctor for this express purpose. Using this drug, like any other drug, requires care and correct understanding of what to expect in light of a full understanding of your own health. Couples and friends sometimes share drugs without the input of their doctor. This is never recommended and is especially unwise during pregnancy.

Is there treatment for an affected baby?

Yes. (Antiviral treatment in general is discussed in chapter 11.) We now have very effective means of killing the virus while it is active. Our problems, in general, in devising new ways to kill herpes are twofold. First, therapy cannot undo damage already done to vital structures, although it can probably stop progression of damage from the infection. Second, it does not alter latent infection (see chapter 1), and therefore virus infection may recur. Suspected neonatal herpes should be quickly and aggressively diagnosed. If a newborn baby becomes ill and the mother has a history of herpes, she should make sure that the pediatrician knows of her history. If the father or any other sexual partner has herpes, that fact is also important, since the mother could then have herpes without knowing it. Remember, too, that neonatal herpes can occur even where both parents have never knowingly had a herpes sore of any kind. Make sure someone explains to you how the possibilities of herpes (and other problems) are being investigated. If herpes is not a consideration to the physician, is that because there is a good reason not to consider it? It is certainly possible to have good medical reasons not to consider the diagnosis of herpes in a newborn, but you should suggest looking for herpes just to make sure that your doctor has thought of the possibility. If your doctor does not consider herpes a possibility, he or she should explain why not.

Adenine arabinoside (ara-A, Vira-A) and acyclovir (Zovirax) are both very useful agents for treating neonatal herpes. Both are effective agents at reducing the disease, regardless of the type of disease at the outset of treatment. Most physicians choose to use acyclovir because it has far fewer side effects and is easier to administer. Neither agent can reverse tissue damage that has already occurred. Physicians' ability to diagnose neonatal herpes more quickly and at much milder stages than in years past is improving the prognosis for newborns quite dramatically. Still, the diagnosis is all too often made after some irreversible harm has already come to the newborn baby. New data also suggest that after a successful initial treatment period with intravenous acyclovir, continuous dosing with oral acyclovir syrup is sometimes recommended after proven neonatal herpes infection, depending on the type and severity of the baby's illness. We need to focus on prevention, but prevention is needed most where it is applied the least-i.e., where the mother does *not* think she has genital herpes.

Occasionally a baby is treated with acyclovir when there is no illness whatsoever, if after a normal vaginal delivery or prolonged membrane rupture it is discovered that the baby has already been exposed. Such a chance exposure to a sore could occur if a sore is noticed only after delivery or in the unlikely event of asymptomatic virus shedding. Although no scientific studies have been performed to support the use of acyclovir in this setting, and many experts in this field prefer not to use the drug in this setting, acyclovir is often used in the newborn if the mother's infection was her first. In a recent report, 12 (46 percent) of 26 newborns who were treated early in infancy and then kept on acyclovir for months after, experienced a reduction in their white blood cell counts. Although this has not been shown to be a clinical problem for the infants, it does point out that the use of any drug, especially in early infancy or childhood, needs to be undertaken only with the careful advice, prescription, and follow-up of a physician. This and other medical issues need to be considered in discussion with your baby's physician. In the future, we may be able to further protect the infant with vaccines for the mother and/or the infant as well as more potent medicines. Even without these safeguards, however, the vast majority of newborn babies of women with recurrent genital herpes do not need any more protection than nature provides.

If I have active herpes during labor, can I have epidural anesthesia? Yes, unless your herpes is a true primary. In that situation, there is a slight risk to the mother of herpes meningitis (see chapter 3), which *might* cause complications from the epidural. In that very unusual case, the anesthetist may wish to opt for a general anesthetic during the cesarean section. Because of this *theoretical risk,* some anesthetists have opted for general anesthetic even during recurrent episodes of genital herpes. Recurrent herpes has never been associated in any way with any proven risk increase after epidural anesthesia. Drs. Ramanathan, Sheth, and Turndorf first published their findings about this in the journal *Anesthesiology* in 1986. They studied 56 women in labor with genital herpes infection, 33 of whom had epidural anesthesia. No complications related to the anesthetic developed in either group. In addition, Drs. Crosby, Halpern, and Rolbin reported their findings in 1989 in the *Canadian Journal of Anaesthesia.* To quote their review of six years' experience in the use of epidural anesthesia at Toronto's Women's College Hospital, "No patient suffered an adverse outcome related to either the anaesthetic or the virus. The theoretical risks of regional anaesthesia in the parturient [woman giving birth 1 with active herpes genitalis are reviewed. We conclude from available data that the risk of an adverse outcome is small and does not contraindicate the use of epidural anaesthesia in patients with recurrent infection." Active recurrent or inactive recurrent genital herpes does not contraindicate epidural anesthesia.

What are my baby's chances of getting herpes?

Neonatal herpes is very unlikely to occur in an infant born to a woman who has genital herpes and knows she has it. By contrast, if the woman does not know she has genital herpes, and especially if the infection occurs for the first time during labor, the baby is at much greater risk. A woman with recurrent infection is unlikely to transmit infection for the following reasons:

1. Any recurrence of herpes is likely to have virus present on the involved area of skin for only a short time. In a closely monitored study in Vancouver, we found that without any special treatment, 50 percent of women with recurrent herpes stopped shedding virus entirely within 56 hours after onset of symptoms. In other words, as soon as virus appears on the skin, nature is already effectively getting rid of it.

2. The mother's immunity to herpes is transferred, in part, to the newborn, offering protection from minor exposure. Babies born to mothers with recurrent herpes have a lot of antibody to herpes. The mother is likely to have high levels of anti-herpes antibody that will be passed on to the baby and the amniotic fluid surrounding the baby, thereby neutralizing the virus in most cases before it has a chance to get into the epithelial cells of the newborn infant.

3. The mother's herpes sore is usually localized, external, and far away from the birth canal, and the cervix is usually free of infection.

4. The mother's recurrent herpes does not make her systemically ill, so the baby is not subject to health problems in the mother.

5. The amount of virus in a recurrent sore is quite small compared with the amount present in primary infection and so is less likely to get to the newborn and cause infection.

6. During primary infection, sores may continue to have active virus present for days or even weeks. Virus in a recurrent sore, however, is present for only a short period of time.

7. The mother has a greater than 95 percent chance of knowing on the basis of her symptoms whether she is culture-positive and potentially exposing the baby. If symptoms of an active phase of infection are present, she will be able to have a cesarean section.

8. Most babies who are exposed to the virus do not actually acquire infection, for the reasons listed above. Of those who do, the vast majority do not develop disease as a result.

9. If exposure to virus has occurred, the physician may choose to treat the baby with a very effective antiviral agent, acyclovir (oral or intravenous). Because the chances of the baby getting sick are so low, even after an episode of obvious exposure to virus, many physicians choose not to use acyclovir. This is an area of academic controversy. I favor treatment before disease develops, in an attempt to prevent this from happening, although I recognize that the clinical trials that have been performed to examine this question are inadequate from the scientific point of view to prove safety and benefit. It may be a very long time before enough patients can be studied to absolutely prove that this approach is beneficial. To me, it just makes clinical sense.

Physicians must make an educated guess that a pregnant woman with recurrent genital herpes will give birth to a baby with a herpes infection, because accurate statistics do not exist. The risk is probably less than one in several thousands that this will happen to any individual with recurrent genital herpes so long as the usual guidelines are followed. The risk of herpes is thus no greater than the risk of a variety of other neonatal diseases. Herpes should not prevent you from having children should you elect to do so.

Crystal ball? In the future, we will probably be suppressing herpes shedding late in pregnancy with safe and effective medications that block the transmission of virus. Screening for herpes will be universal, not limited to women who know they have herpes. Women who are at risk of getting herpes during pregnancy will be protected by vaccine taken before conception or possibly during pregnancy. Where it is not known if the woman is at risk, and thus the neonate may be at risk, the baby will be vaccinated to prevent infection at birth.

Herpes and Cancer

Are herpes and cancer related?

Although some of the human herpes viruses do cause cancer, there is no proof that herpes simplex does. A scientific argument about the causes of cervical cancer still exists, however. Let us review the evidence. First of all, did you know that sex causes cancer? This is not even controversial. Sex is associated with cancers that result from the transmission of human immunodeficiency virus (HIV). People with HIV who develop AIDS quite frequently develop cancers as a result of their immunodeficiency. These cancers include Kaposi's sarcoma (caused by human herpes virus type 8), lymphoma, and certain squamous cell cancers. In some cases, the cause of an AIDS-related tumor is infection, in that the immunodeficiency has reduced the person's ability to fight the infection normally in order to prevent the cancer.

Even without the transmission of HIV, however, sex is associated with cancer of the cervix and of the vulva. Cancer of the cervix is a common tumor in prostitutes, rare in Catholic nuns. It occurs more often in women who begin having first sexual contact early and who have more sexual partners. It is not surprising, then, to find that one sexually transmitted agent, namely herpes simplex, is more common in women with cervical cancer than in those without. About twenty-five years ago, studies began to show over and over again a *seroepidemiologic* association between the two diseases. This means that a blood, or serum ("sero-"), test for antibodies to herpes simplex type 2 is positive more often in groups ("-epidemiologic") of women *with* cancer than in groups without. By themselves, however, these studies tell us little. Sex causes cervical cancer. Furthermore, sex predisposes an individual to getting genital herpes. So it is no surprise to find that both herpes and cancer of the cervix have been found to be more common in women who have more sex-related risk factors. It would have been more surprising not to find this.

The *human papillomavirus* (HPV) , known to cause venereal warts, has also been called an *oncogenic* (cancer-causing) virus. Evidence now overwhelmingly points to this virus as the true cervical cancer virus. Certain subtypes are very closely related to cancer development.

As we get better and better at detecting and probing for causes, invasive cancer of the cervix is becoming less and less common. Early Pap smear changes are often treated so quickly that cancer is never allowed to develop.

The Pap smear is an important health tool for any woman who has been sexually active. Early detection means that cervical cancer is unlikely to develop, and an abnormality is very easy to detect before it becomes cancerous. If cancer does develop, it starts out very slowly, allowing lots of time to take successful curative action during the early stages. The Pap smear is used for detection-use it regularly.

Cancer of the vulva, the woman's external genitals, is also a slow-growing cancer. It is much less common than cancer of the cervix. It is now also known to be caused by human papillomavirus. The symptoms are commonly external itching, pain, or the observance of a growth. Its most common locations-on the external genitals-parallel those of genital herpes. Although itching of the vaginal area is seldom related to cancer, persistent vaginal itching should be explored for possible causes. See your physician if you are concerned.

If I have herpes, is it on the cervix? Inside the vagina?

During primary genital herpes, nine out of ten women with herpes on the labia also have herpes on the cervix. Sometimes this may cause *cervicitis,* or inflammation of the cervix with an associated vaginal discharge. Sores can develop on the cervix as well. Herpes is probably a cause of nonspecific cervicitis more often than is realized. Cervicitis and discharge are common during primary herpes, even in the absence of external sores-sometimes because external sores develop a bit later in the course of infection and sometimes because external sores never develop during primary herpes.

During recurrences of genital herpes, herpes on the cervix is uncommon. A carefully performed study has shown that herpes can be recovered from the cervix in only 4 percent of recurrent cases. In fact, it may be that many of these were not really on the cervix but appeared to be there because of the "wet path" that exists between cervix and sore. It is impossible to examine the cervix without first touching the vulva and entrance to the vagina-typical external areas of recurrent infection. Genital herpes is an external infection for the most part. In women, it occurs mainly on the vaginal lips, the perianal area, the perineum (between anus and vagina) and the pubic region. The cervix is an uncommon site of infection during recurrences.

What are my chances of getting cervical cancer?

There are different degrees of cervical cancer, according to epidemiologists who look at the problem and according to the women affected by this disease. Cancer detected on a Pap smear before any damage whatsoever is done to the person occurs in about 1 in 1,000 women over the age of twenty. Depending on the study, the risk increases to 2 to 8 per 1,000 women with genital herpes. Other factors, such as smoking cigarettes may also increase the risk of developing cancer of the cervix. Clinically significant cervical cancer (one that has gone far enough that it might do harm to the person if not dealt with immediately) occurs with much less frequency (closer to 7 or 8 of 100,000 women over the age of twenty). The risk of this type of cancer occurring in people with genital herpes increases to approximately 15 to 100 cases per 100,000 women over the age of twenty probably because, overall, people with herpes are statistically more likely to also have infection with human papillomavirus. The average age of occurrence is the late forties, although cervical cancer can be seen as early as the teens or as late as the eighties. The responsible virus is not herpes. But people who have herpes also have human papillomavirus more than other people do.

What should I do to prevent cervical cancer from becoming a problem?

A *Pap smear* is a simple procedure and should be part of your annual gynecological examination. It is quick and simple to do correctly. The best time to have it done is just before or at ovulation, when estrogen hormone levels are high and the cells are flatter and easier to interpret under the microscope. The test can also be done at any other time if ovulation is an inconvenient time to make the visit to the physician. First, a plastic or metal speculum is inserted into the vagina, as pictured in figure 10. This allows the examiner to see the cervix by gently pushing the walls of the vagina aside. Any vaginal discharge and cervical mucus coating the cervix are then swabbed away using a cotton swab. A wooden scraper shaped like a stretched Popsicle stick is used to scrape cells from the surface of the cervix onto a slide, which is then sent to the laboratory.

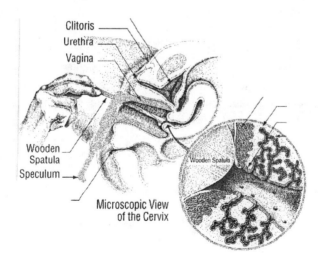

The Pap smear detects any unusual cells from the cervix. If cells are cancerous, it will detect them. If cells are just upset from infection, it will detect them also. All of these cells will be called abnormal. Since cancer of the cervix is very slow to grow, a yearly Pap smear is an adequate test. Some physicians feel that Pap smears are needed less frequently. As long as they stay normal-Class lone per year is plenty. If your Pap smear is abnormal in any way, more frequent smears may be appropriate. If you have had several normal Pap smears on a yearly basis and you are not changing sexual partners and your sexual partner is not changing sexual partners, then it may be appropriate to have Pap smears performed less often. Discuss these issues with your physician.

Whether you have herpes or not, the yearly Pap smear is a good idea however. Rest assured that if you follow this regimen, any detected cancer of the cervix is likely to be curable. I recommend putting this cancer issue out of your mind except for one big red mark on each new calendar-the day for your yearly Pap test.

My Pap smear is abnormal. What does that mean?

The Pap smear is a method of examining the cells that line the cervix. Anything that changes those cells will change your Pap smear. During primary herpes, a Pap smear is abnormal from infection but changes back to normal after the primary episode has cleared; this abnormal smear is of no concern. Other infectionssuch as *trichomoniasis, bacterial oaginosis,* and *gonorrhea-may* also change the Pap smear. In each case, if the Pap has become abnormal as a symptom of infection, treatment of the infection will cause the Pap to revert to normal eventually. A Pap will also be abnormal if cancer of the cervix has developed. It is obviously important to find out if your abnormal Pap is from infection or cancer. How is this done?

Pap abnormalities are classified. The classifications vary from city to city, state to state, province to province, and country to country. There are scores ranging from normal to obvious invasive cancer, with many gray areas in between. If the score is abnormal, there are several things to do. If the most severely abnormal condition is detected, indicating invasive cancer, a *colposcopy* is gen-

136

erally performed. If a less severely abnormal condition is discovered, your best bet is first to make sure that all possible infections have been ruled out. Your doctor will do (or may already have done) a culture test for Chlamydia, gonorrhea, and Candida. A microscopic examination for *Trichomonas uagina/is* and an assessment for bacterial vaginosis are also performed. If your abnormal Pap was taken during or shortly after your primary herpes, you may also want to repeat the test to see if the situation has improved on its own. If another infection is present, have the Pap test done again two or three months later to see if it has returned to normal.

Let's say you still have an abnormal test. If an infection was present, you've had it treated. You've waited several months. If the score shows only a mild abnormality, you will likely be advised to wait and see and to have another test in a few months. Probably, this abnormal score will eventually vanish. If your score shows consistently abnormal cells, you may be sent for a colposcopy test. This is an examination of the cervix much like the Pap smear. The speculum exam is repeated, as for the Pap smear. Then the physician inserts a microscope-like instrument through the speculum to take a very close look at the surface of the cervix. Biopsies are taken for further laboratory examination. A biopsy of the cervix may feel like a pinch or may not be felt at all. The procedure is very, very safe. A small amount of bleeding is to be expected. The laboratory examines the biopsies and offers an opinion. If invasive or microinvasive cancer is present on a biopsy, the therapy is removal of the cancer. Surgery may be required. The most common surgery is the *cone biopsy,* in which only the inner core of the cervix is removed through the vagina. Generally, a cone biopsy does not prevent either sexual intercourse or normal birth.

The different possible therapies to be chosen at this point are beyond the scope of this book. If your biopsy is in a less severe category, arguments exist about what therapy you should have. You may be advised in one center to have a cone biopsy for severe dysplasia (abnormal tissue growth), and in another center to wait, see, and repeat for *carcinoma in situ.* Why all the conflicting advice? Most cervices in this gray area will not progress to invasive cancer, if left alone. Many will revert to a normal condition with no intervention. However, many physicians argue that most is not good enough.

The safest (and most invasive) thing to do with cervical tissue diagnosed as being in a gray area is to remove it from the cervix. Have you ever been asked if you see the proverbial glass of water as half full or half empty? The right course of action is not cast in stone: if the situation should arise, discuss it at length with your doctor and read a lot more on the topic. Keep in mind that if you have an abnormal result from a routine Pap smear, you have found the problem early and can get treatment that is effective and safe!

Printed in the United States
145669LV00002B/83/P